Healing Yourself with Vegetables

Natural Remedies for a Healthier You

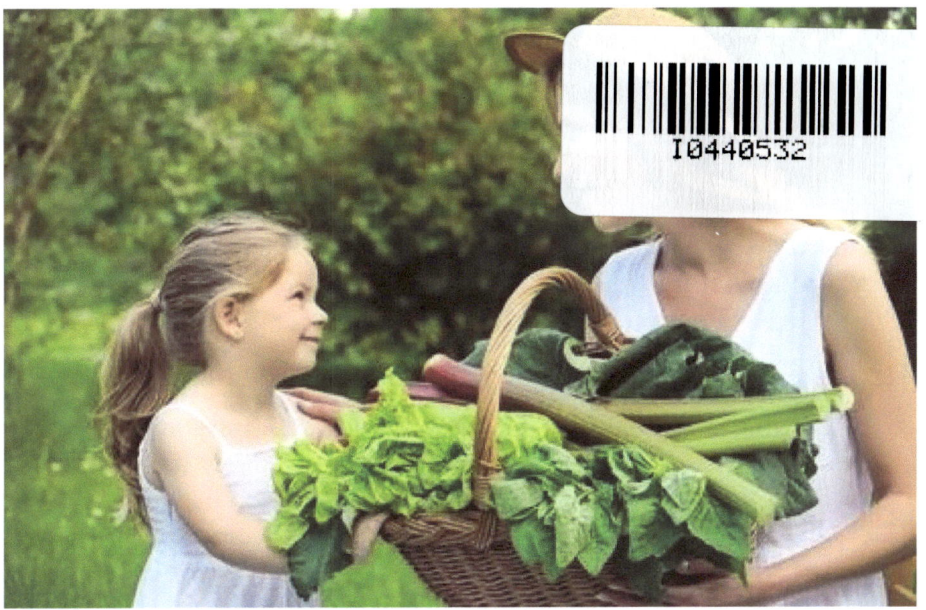

Dueep Jyot Singh

Healthy Living Series

Mendon Cottage Books

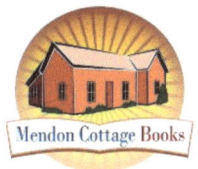

JD-Biz Publishing

Our books are available at

1. Amazon.com
2. Barnes and Noble
3. Itunes
4. Kobo
5. Smashwords
6. Google Play Books

Table of Contents

Introduction

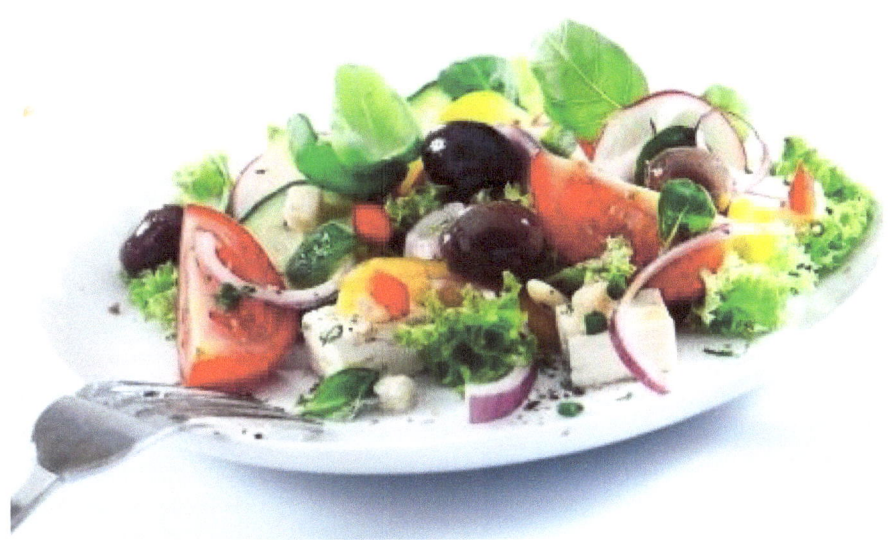

I wrote a book on healing yourself naturally named **Healing Yourself with Fruit** – Click here to download and this is the next part of the series. Here you are going to learn how to cure yourselves naturally with the help of vegetables which you can find very easily.

It is a well-known fact that in ancient times, people who were really ill were taken out of the city or from the tribe to a little Hermitage, on the outskirts of the area. They were then put in the hands of the wise men, of the land. These wise men were then given plenty of opportunity in order to experiment on their patients.

With the passing of years, they soon found out that there were some vegetables, herbs, spices, and fruit, which could cure a number of ailments. Naturally, all this was done through trial and error in the initial stages.

That is because these vegetables have a number of essential minerals and nutrients, which are necessary to keep the body healthy. So this book is going to tell you about some of the easily available vegetables, which are going to help in the curing of a large number of ailments.

How to Use Vegetables Effectively

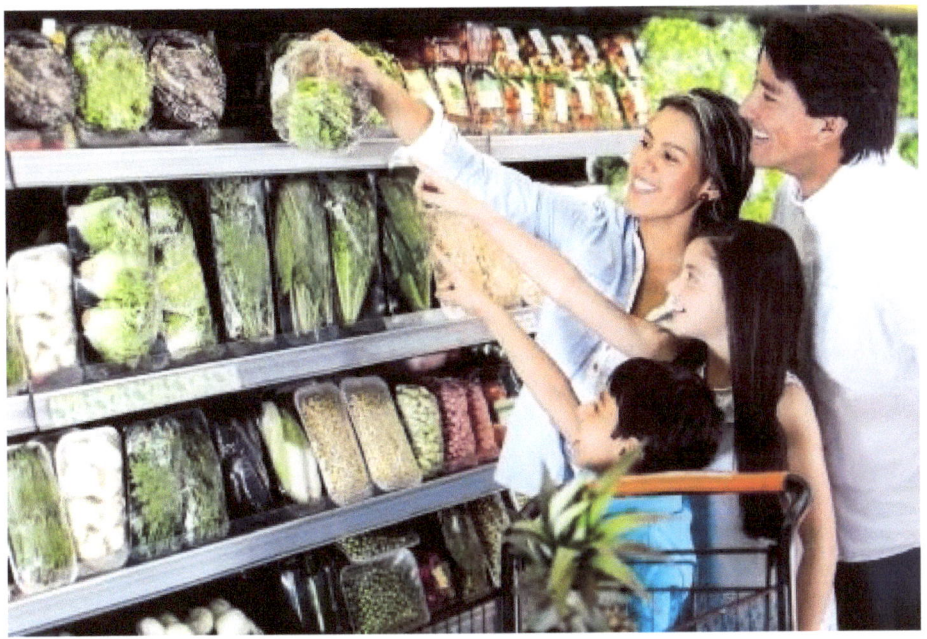

Most of us are so used to going into the vegetable section of our supermarket and picking up all the different packets there. According to us, they are fresh, because they have just been stocked in the shelves that morning. However, packaging causes many of these vegetables to grow stale with the passing of time.

If we are lucky enough to have a kitchen garden in which we are growing a large number of vegetables, we are going to have a really good supply of fresh, leafy and green vegetables to add to our daily diet. These are going to take care of all the bio physiological functions of our body and make sure that it works in a proper and naturally healthy manner.

So when you are getting ready to select vegetables, make sure that they are fresh, green, leafy, and full of fibers. I remember a joke about a young man watching a lady, old enough to be his grandmother, in the vegetable section, searching for a cabbage. He kept waiting till she had chosen the best cabbage in the lot, and then he asked her politely, "Ma'am, now could you please pick out the second best cabbage for me?"

This might be an amusing joke, but here you see a very practical point. The lady was taking her time to choose a cabbage which was fresh, green, leafy, and crisp. She knew that her chosen vegetable was not going to have marks of disease or fungal spots.

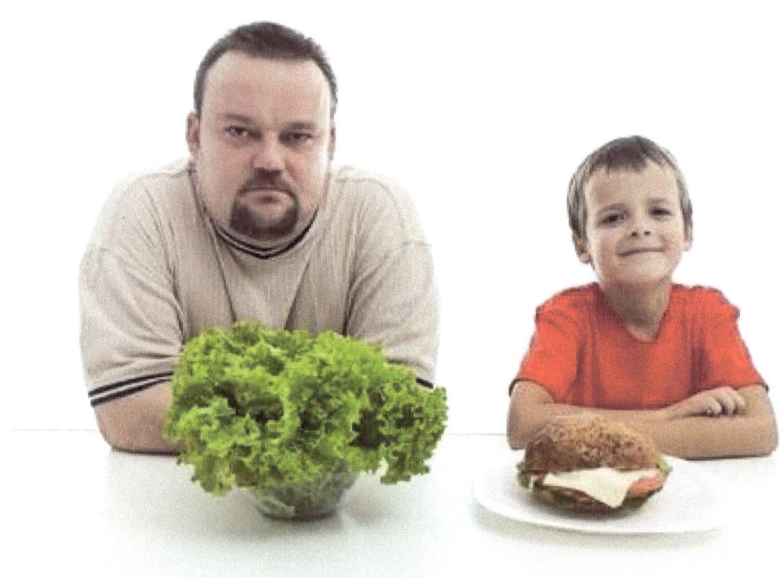

When we were kids and were learning to appreciate good food, there were times when we preferred meat to vegetables. Our father knew that just telling us to "Eat up your vegetables, they are good for you" would immediately put our backs up and we would never eat them again, just because we were born stubborn, managed to make us interested in vegetables by a simple expedient story.

According to him, green and leafy vegetables were the cleaning up agents in our stomach. For example, the seeds in the okra were rollers, just like the roller bearings in our roller – skates. They went rolling in our stomach, gathering all the best material, and pushing them out. That was the reason why we never suffered from constipation.

We loved this explanation. And that is why we loved all the vegetables, especially those with "rollers".

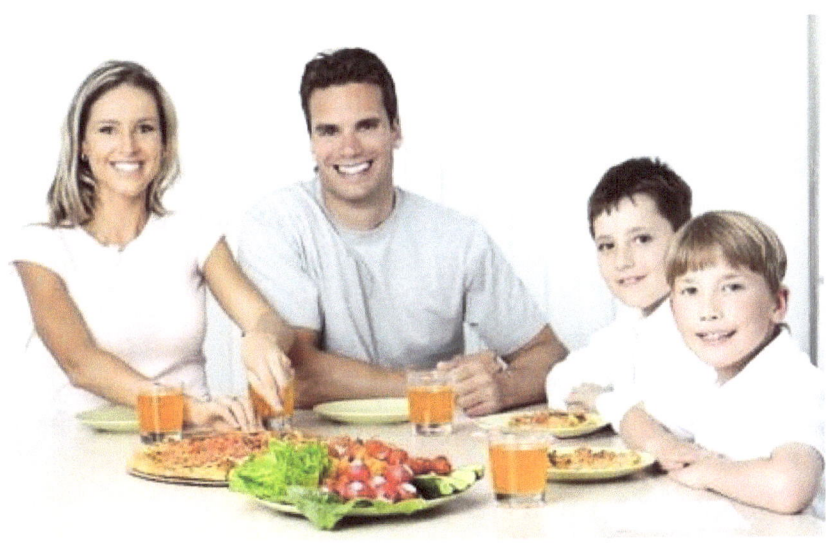

You cannot use any other food item or chemically manufactured supplement as a substitute for healthy, leafy and fresh vegetables. Apart from imparting lots of variety and taste to your food, these vegetables help in the manufacture of digestive juices, speeding up your metabolism and circulatory system, strengthening your immunity system, rectifying your digestive system and adding to your state of good health.

Also, according to father, the rest of the vegetables were capable of producing a lot of bulk in your tummy, and getting rid of all the digested accumulated waste. This explanation sounded very logical to us children, because according to him, the more vegetables we ate, the more "bulk" we had in our stomachs, which had to be eliminated.

And because we did not suffer from any constipation, we had clear skins, a healthy Constitution, excellent powers of concentration, lots of energy, and a very cheerful positive physical, spiritual, mental and emotional outlook. The last one may not have been a direct effect of vegetables, but more of our up – bringing, but a healthy body meant a healthy mind.

So here are some common sense and useful tips, which you need to implement whenever you go out to gather those green leafy vegetables unto you.

If the leaves are very green and leafy, they are going to wilt foster, when compared to vegetables which are not leafy. That is why it is more sensible to use them right away, rather than wrapping them up in wet cloth and putting them in the fridge.

We have a weekly farmers market in our area every Friday. That is the time when the people in our neighborhood and beyond visit this large market and choose vegetables for the rest of the week. Tomatoes and potatoes can be preserved till next Friday, but spinach, cabbages, lettuce and other green leafy vegetables are bought to be eaten within the next two days, in salads or cooked.

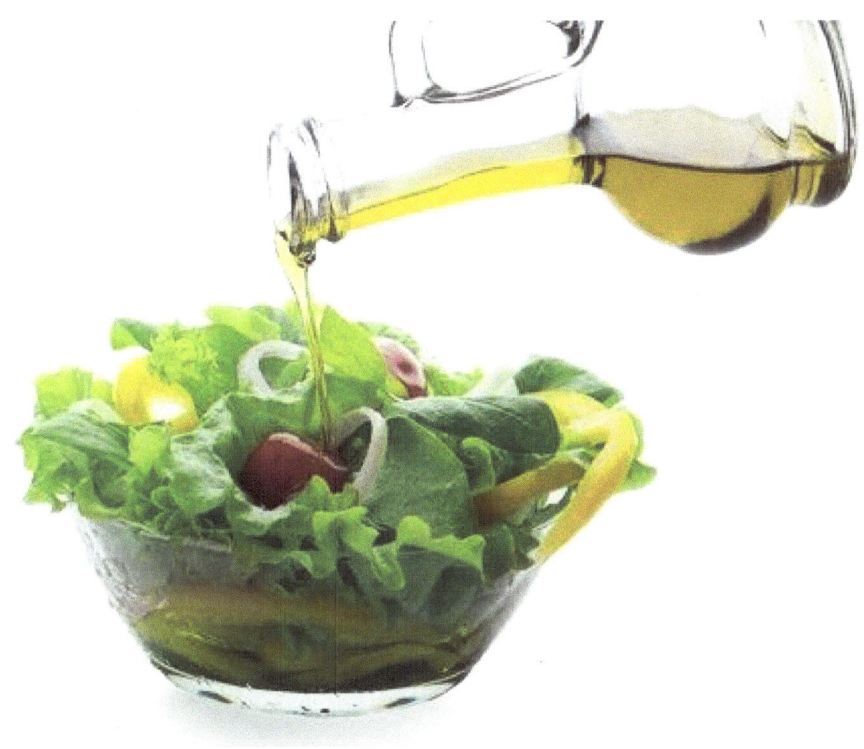

The best thing about this farmers market is that we do not have to bother about the middlemen. The prices are fixed early in the morning, and by night time, they are reduced to about 80% of the morning's price because the farmers do not want to take their vegetables back home in their tractors and trucks.

I was astonished to see a farmer dumping his stock of tomatoes on the road, a couple of months ago. One only has to blame the country's or state's government for this state of affairs, because there was no way in which the farmers in our State could send their excess glut of tomatoes to other States or even export them abroad. They did not have the infrastructure, nor the know-how. And this is the 21st-century!

So these vegetables were dumped on the road. And they rotted there, because the people of our State were too dignified to pick up free vegetables from off the streets.

What a pity, I told myself. A little bit of sense and application, and all these tomatoes could be turned by the family members of the farmers into local produce like sauces and chutneys. But one would rather dump vegetables on the road, then do something constructive and prosperous which entails a little bit of hard work.

So next time you get the vegetables of your choice, just wipe them with a clean cloth to get rid of the dust. You are going to wash them, only before you cook them. Continuous washing is going to get rid of all the essential nutrients below the surface of the skin.

Radish leaves, tomatoes, carrots and beetroots should be eaten raw, as far as possible. The more you chew them, the more they are going to help aid in the digestion because when they are mixed up with the saliva, they become very powerful digestive agents.

As kids, we were not encouraged to eat between meals, but our meals always had carrots and tomatoes and other green leafy vegetables as salads. These vegetables were freshly obtained from the garden, and fed to us within the hour. We were told to munch the carrots as often as we could, because that exercise would strengthen our teeth, gums and jaws. It did! Much better than chewing gum and healthier.

Look at all the traditional cuisines, modern and ancient. Food is always served fresh, after it has been cooked with care. In ancient times, the members of the family were so hungry that they finished up every meal. At that time, the amount of food was also limited, and it was very rare that food would be left over for another helping at the next meal time.

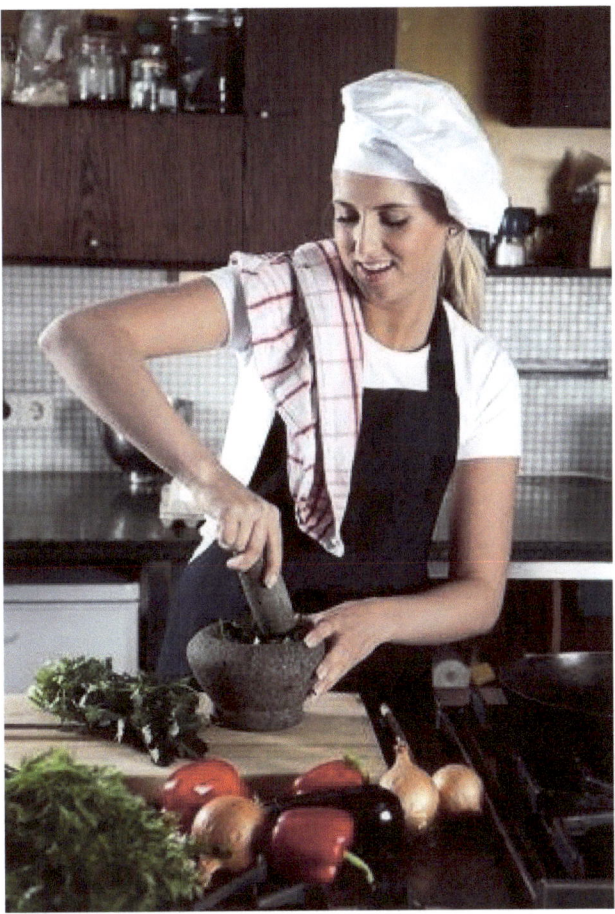

That is why everything was cooked fresh and fed fresh. But thanks to the preservative methods of the modern age, the lady of the house cooks just once in the morning, and the whole family is going to eat this food throughout the rest of the day. Some ladies cook just once a week, and put the food items away in the freezer to be defrosted when needed.

That is perhaps we are more bothered about expediency and time-saving than in eating freshly cooked food at the right time. So as far as possible, eat your fresh meal, within two – three hours and try not to put the leftovers in the fridge.

However, if it is necessary for you to preserve some green leafy vegetables, wrap them up in a wet paper – not a print paper – until it is airtight. You can also use airtight polythene bags. I have found a number of vegetable bags being sold by a large number of suppliers globally which are made up of a mixture of polythene, polyester and cloth. These are very sturdy and I have managed to keep vegetables in them for about four – five days, when I could not cook them right away.

http://www.amazon.com/flip-tumble-Reusable-Produce-Bags/dp/B002UXQ7QQ/ref=sr_1_2?ie=UTF8&qid=1443335251&sr=8-2&keywords=Vegetables+storage+mesh+bags

I found these rates very exorbitant, but you can always look for bargains now that you know what to look for, in your choice of polyester or cotton mesh bags.

Spinach

Just like Popeye, I like spinach. That is because I was lucky enough to have a good cook cooking spinach for me, when I was a child. Many times, children do not like to eat food, because the food served to them is unappetizing, bland, boring, or even tasteless and soggy.

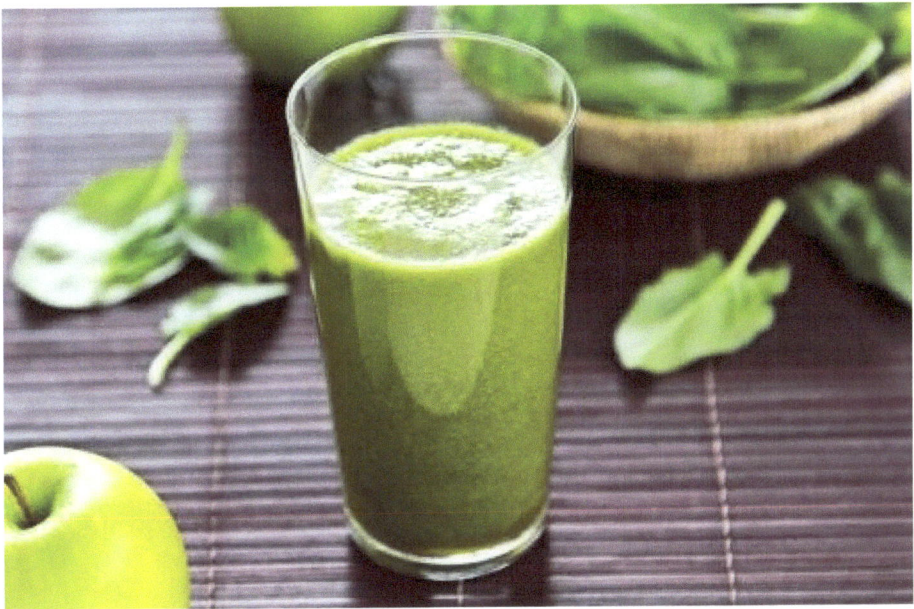

I remember going to a relative's house where she had just cooked spinach for the family. The spinach was watery, and totally unappealing. I just looked at it and wondered where the delicious spinach of my childhood had gone? Her family did not touch the spinach nor the soggy okra, nor the bland mashed potatoes. They made do with bread-and-butter.

So if you are one of those could not care less moms, who could not feed delicious, appetizing and healthy nourishing meals to her kids, please wake up. It is not too late. Your children are being deprived of healthy nutrients, minerals, carbohydrates, fats, proteins, and vitamins, because you have been feeding them junk food or TV dinners.

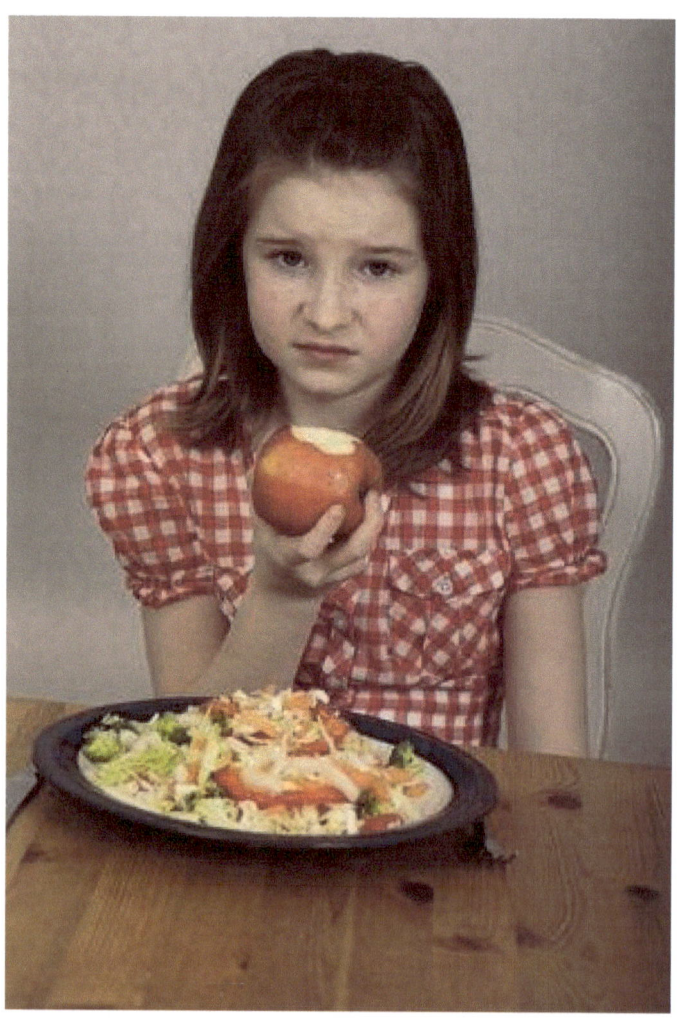

And because you did not teach them to appreciate vegetables and fruit, when they were young, this is what you are going to face whenever you give them greens to eat.

Anyway, coming back to spinach. If you have to boil it before you cook it, just add a little bit of salt to the boiling water. This is going to preserve the green color, instead of turning it yellowish olive green after the spinach leaves have been boiled. Use just about four tablespoons full of water, for boiling, mildly, because the spinach leaves are going to produce enough of water, the moment they are subjected to heat. This boiling is done on low heat.

Spinach is nature's mine for iron. People suffering from anemia are encouraged to eat lots and lots of spinach, because they are going to get more red blood corpuscles growing thanks to this iron content. You cannot eat iron in its natural form, so that is why nature has managed to incorporate this trace elements in vegetables. In fact, it also has a lot of sodium in it, so you need not put extra salt for sodium content when you are cooking spinach.

Spinach for Stones

If you are suffering from any sort of stones, including gallbladder stones and kidney stones, here is an excellent remedy which is going to get rid of the stones in three days. But that is because this is a drastic cure with lots of spinach and radishes. You will need 200 g of fresh spinach juice which will need to be fed to the patient four times a day. After each two doses of spinach, you will have to give the patient hundred grams of radish juice. That means six doses in all, of two juices, and 24 doses in three days.

Gallstones

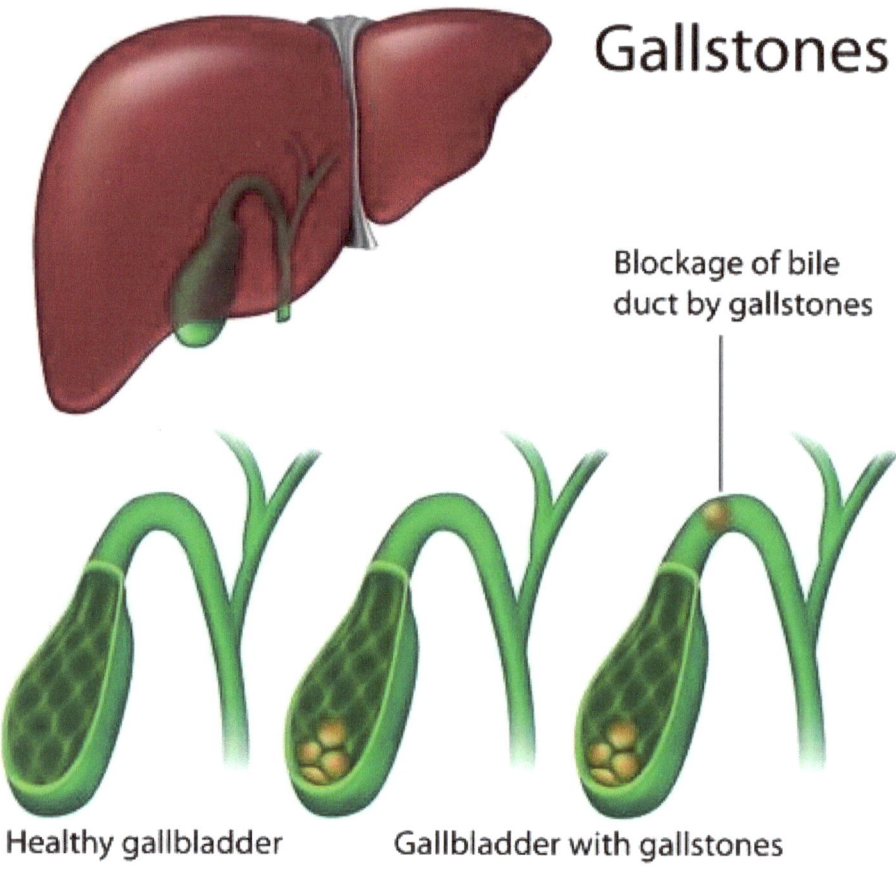

Blockage of bile
duct by gallstones

Healthy gallbladder   Gallbladder with gallstones

No wonder those gallstones want out with all that onslaught of spinach and radishes.

Turnips

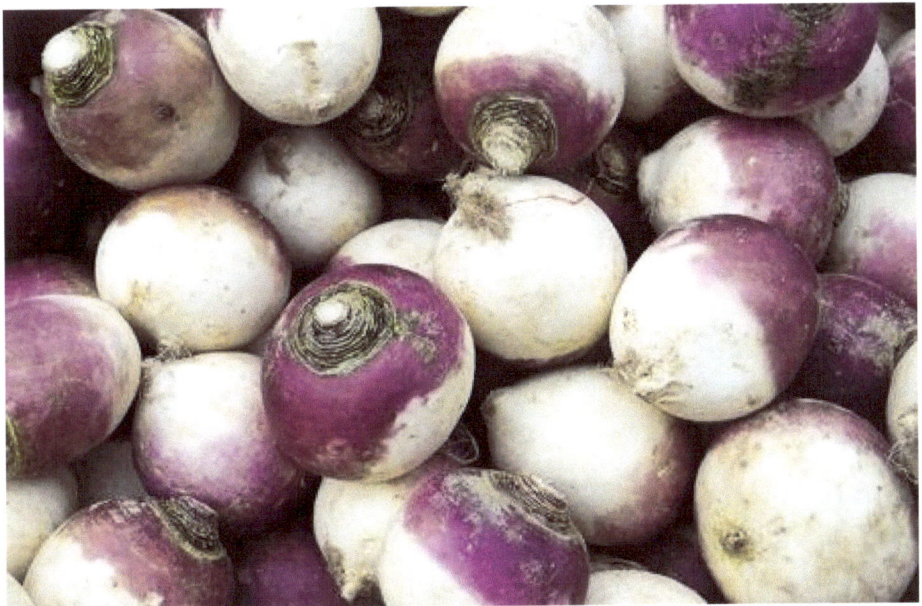

Turnips were such an integral part of mankind's diet down the ages, that many ancient fairytales always have the farmers working in their turnip fields when they either confront an ogre, or a bear or a fairy.

Turnips for Your Teeth

Eat a raw turnip every morning, after you have brushed your teeth. This is capable of giving your teeth a real shine as well as keeping them healthy. Also, these turnips prevent any sort of bleeding from your gums. The best part is, that you are eating them raw, and adding lots of nutrients to your system.

Diabetes

People suffering from diabetes are going to find a visible relief through eating turnips. Turnips are found easily in the winter. So dry them in the sun, so that you can eat them throughout the rest of the year. The sun-dried turnips should be boiled, so that they can turn soft before eating.

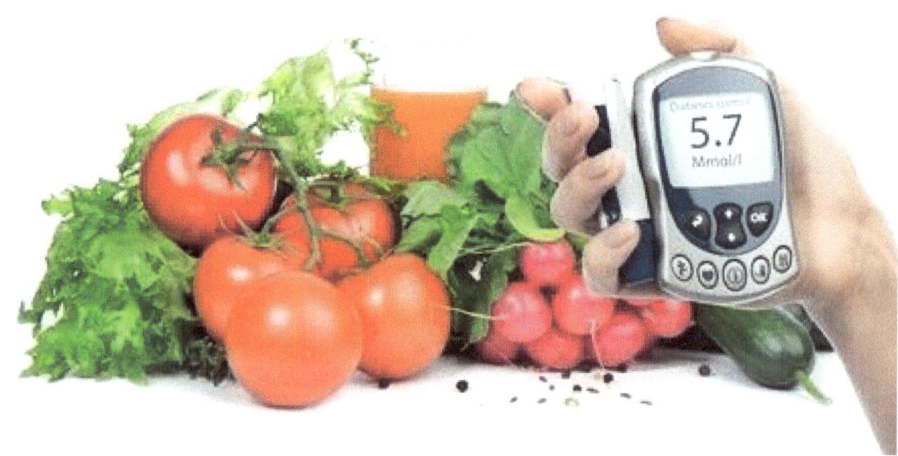

Kidney Stones and Gallbladder Stones

According to ancient medical treatises, turnips were used to cure stones in the gallbladder and in the kidney. This was done by mixing 20 g each of carrot seeds and turnip seeds. After that, a radish was hollowed out and the pulp removed from inside. These seeds were then placed inside the radish covering and roasted over an open fire, especially coals. That was the cooking procedure, followed for millenniums, down the ages and roasting on coals is still a favorite way of cooking food in many parts of the world today.

When you have roasted the radish, so take out the seeds and grind them. Now you are going to take one teaspoonful of these seeds morning and evening with water. This has to be done for one month because this is a long-term natural cure getting rid of the stones inside. You are going to be cured in one month. This is a time-tested remedy.

Pumpkins

Peter Peter pumpkin eater could not do without pumpkins, even though many people think it a boring vegetable to eat. But they do not know that a large number of vegetarians all over the world managed to get their carbohydrates through pumpkins and potatoes. Pumpkins also have a large number of essential nutrients and minerals which are necessary to keep your body functioning properly.

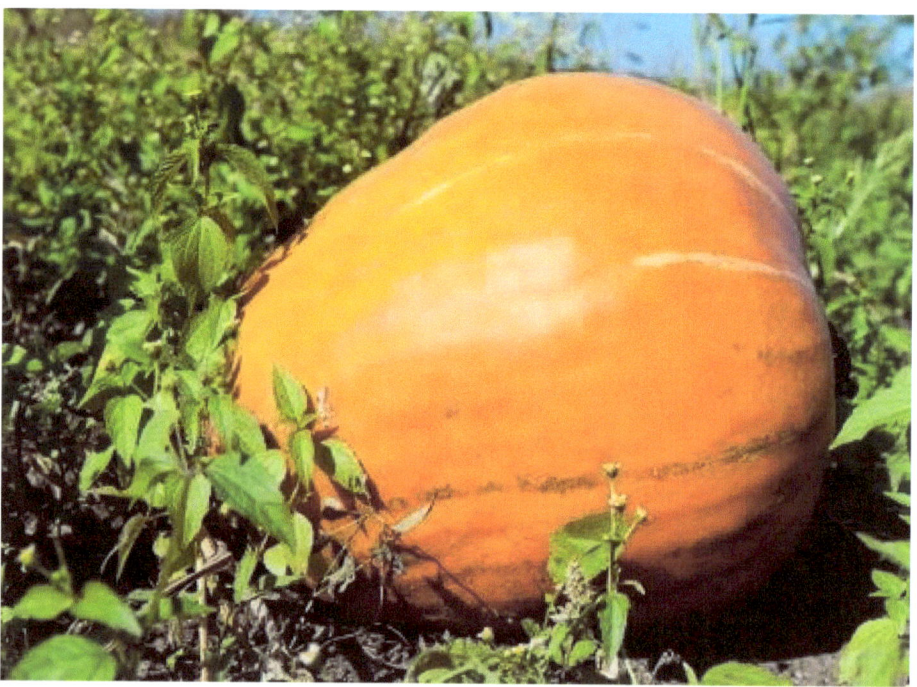

However, pumpkins have had a bad PR down the ages, because like beans, they are considered to be capable of producing flatulence. So the next time you cook pumpkins, just add some fenugreek seeds to the cooking mixture. You are not going to suffer from any flatulence ever.

If you are feeling lethargic and do not have too much of energy, here is a suggestion – make up a mixture of ground pumpkin and mustard leaves with a little bit of mustard seeds and fenugreek seeds. Mix it in yogurt, add your preferred spices, salt-and-pepper, and cayenne pepper and eat this dip/salad/nourishing accompaniment. You are going to find yourself revitalized.

Tomatoes

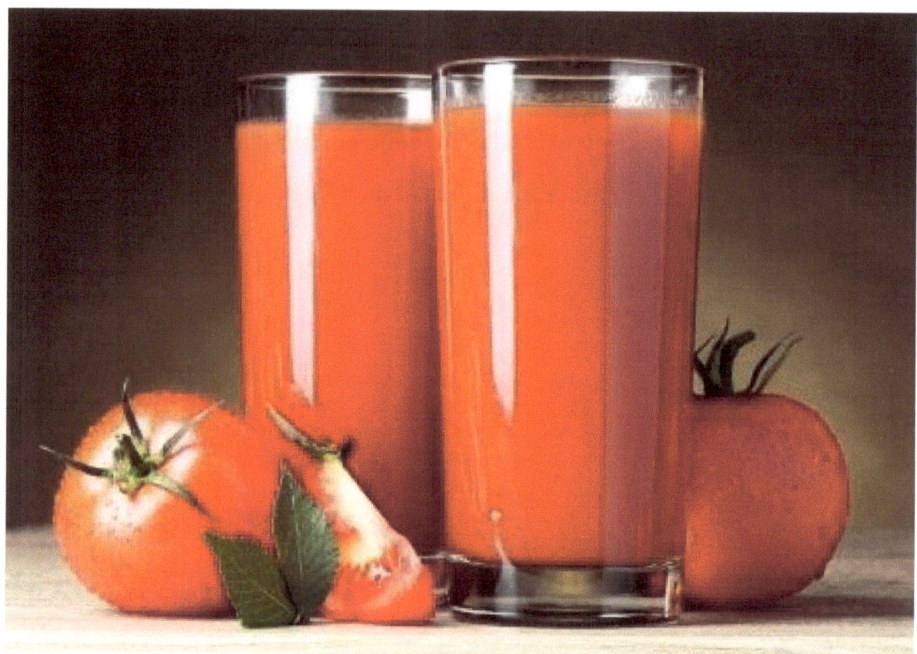

It is surprising to know that tomatoes were not known extensively in the ancient world, until more than 600 years ago. In the same way, chilies came to the East from the West in the 14th century. But chilies as well as tomatoes have become so incorporated in Easton cuisine, that one cannot imagine any meal without chunks of tomatoes, fried, roasted, boiled, or minced added to the meal, during cooking.

Nevertheless, let me tell you this strange story about tomatoes. In many parts of the East, it was not eaten because it was colored the color of blood. In the same way more than 200 years ago, American pioneers would not touch tomatoes, because they thought them poisonous. Nevertheless, tomatoes have managed to survive as a part of our daily diet. Adding lots of tomatoes to your diet – remove the seeds first – keeps your system healthy.

People suffering from kidney problems may have been eating lots of tomato seeds. The pulp without seeds keeps your kidneys healthy. However, tomato seeds collecting in your stomach are capable of causing stones. But that is only going to happen, if you are already suffering from stones. Nevertheless, remove the seeds before eating. Why take chances? And if you do not want to do that, remember to drink lots of water, when you are eating tomatoes.

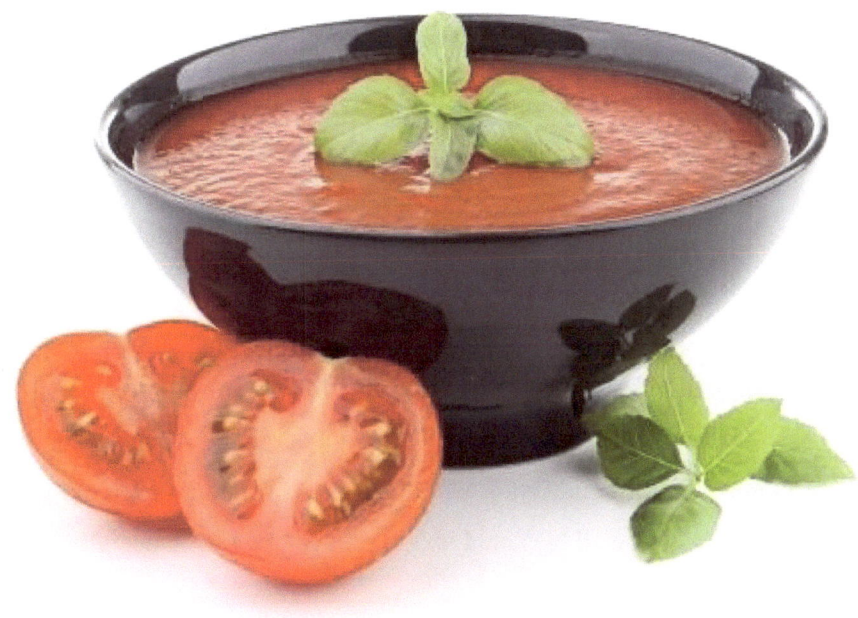

Night Blindness

Tomatoes are an excellent source of potassium. That is why they are good for your eyes. In fact, in ancient times, people suffering from night blindness were fed lots of seedless tomatoes, raw. So they managed to get their needed supplement of vitamin A necessary to cure night blindness.

The method of doing that was of cutting the pulp, getting rid of the seeds and then chewing on the pulp to obtain the juice. Swallow the juice first. Then swallow the pulp. You could also try a mixture of tomato juice and carrot juice to get rid of night blindness.

For Blemishes

Here is a beauty remedy, which is going to help people suffering from skin problems, blemishes, and sunburn. Just chop up a piece of tomato, to cover that affected area. Leave it overnight. Do this for one week. Your skin is going to come back to its natural color, while getting rid of the black marks, blemishes and skin burn.

Nausea

If you are suffering from any sort of nausea, all you have to do is cut a tomato into small pieces, deseed it, mix it well with pepper, rock salt and lemon juice. Sniff it before you eat it! You could also sniff a mixture of tomato pieces with fresh mint leaves before you eat them. Also, tomato juice with mint leaves, pepper and rock salt along with a little bit of lemon juice is excellent to keep you well hydrated and to prevent nausea, especially during the summer.

Drinking lots of fresh tomato juice is excellent for your teeth. Try it out. Tomato juice is also excellent for constipation.

Diabetes Cure

Also, here is a suggestion for people suffering from diabetes. Drink plenty of tomato soup, with the seeds removed. You may also want to add the juice of bitter gourds, to this mixture. Drink it for one month with every meal. And then look at the difference. And then recommend this to all your friends suffering from diabetes.

Digestive Problems

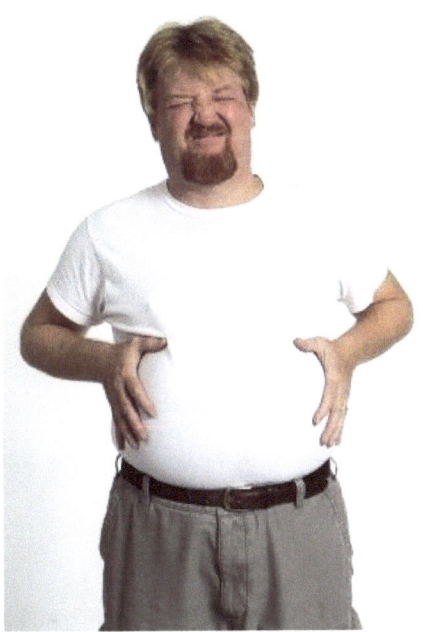

There is a digestive ailment, where people are not capable of digesting their food properly. That is why they eat in very small quantities. However, even that food is not digested, giving rise to heaviness in the stomach and in the head, a feeling of nausea, lethargy, and other digestion ailment related side effects.

Under such circumstances, you need to eat lots of deseeded tomatoes with pepper and rock salt. The more you eat, the better your digestive system is going to perk up.

Dry Skin

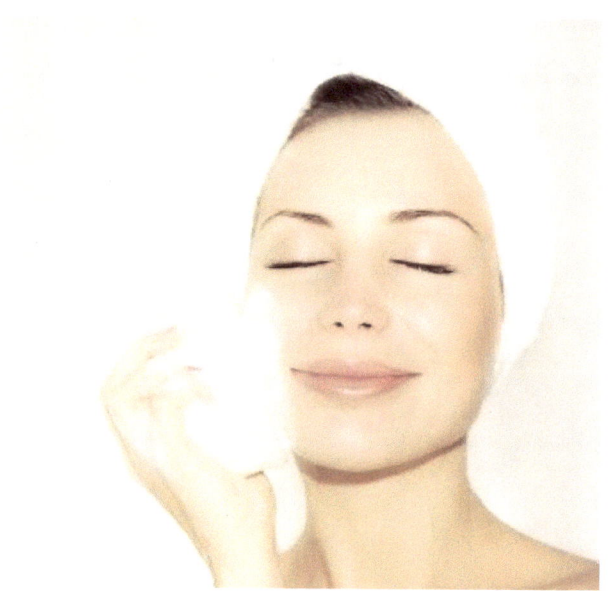

Dry skin can be prevented with lots of fresh tomato juice.

This is one remedy which has been forgotten down the ages, but here it is again. If you are suffering from dry skin and want it to be restored to its previous state of silky good health, just drink plenty of fresh tomato juice – deseeded – morning and night. In the winter, you can add a little bit of warm water to this mixture.

Apart from this, you can mix 10 g tomato juice in 20 g of your favorite massage oil, and apply it all over the affected areas. Allow the oil to assimilate for half an hour, and then shower. Your skin is going to reach its state of soft silkiness in two days.

Tuberculosis

Tuberculosis was once upon a time, one of the most prolific of killers all over the world. However, today, thanks to the number of drugs available to us, it is not such a scary disease anymore. Nevertheless, if you are in an area where there is a person suffering from tuberculosis and you do not have access to any drugs, you are going to cure him with this natural cure, which was used when there were no antibiotics or drugs around for millenniums.

You are going to give the patient 15 g of tomato juice – without seeds – in which you have put hundred grams of cod liver oil. Give it to the patient once a day, for two months. You are going to see him start recuperating within one month itself. After one month, you are going to reduce the quantities into half. That means 50 g of oil and 7 g of juice for the next one month. And whatever the protesting and unbelieving doctors, researchers and scientists may say, the patient is going to be thoroughly cured within two months.

White Spots on Skin – vitiligo

These spots normally occur on portions of your body, where the melanin has disappeared due to some reason. In Eastern medicine, the reason is supposed to be a deficiency of calcium. This can be removed by eating a mixture of tomato and coconuts.

I asked one of my friends, living in an area by the seaside, where coconuts were in abundance, whether this cure was true. She said yes. And because her diet consisted of lots of coconuts along with tomatoes, she would always have a clear and healthy complexion with absolutely no patchy white spots caused due to a melanin deficiency.

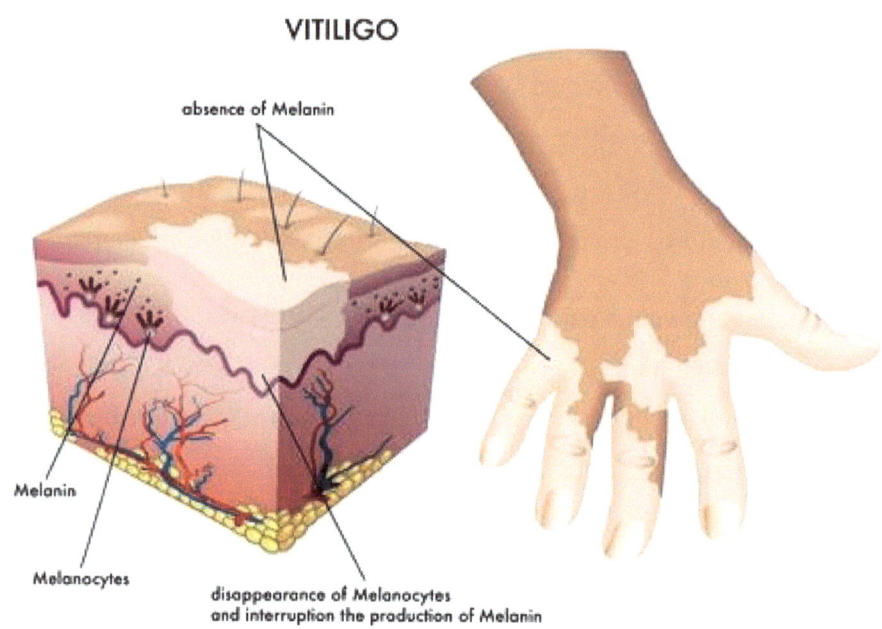

Anybody suffering from these white spots just had to cure himself internally with coconut and tomato and put on a piece of tomato pulp on that spot at night and tie it. In the morning, one had to have a bath without any soap. This would bring the skin color back to normal.

Seriously, I tried this out three days ago, when I was shocked to see the skin underneath my eyes bleaching out to white, instead of its normal dusky hue. I was not going to have white marks under my eyes, in the pouch area, where I have seen them in a number of persons.

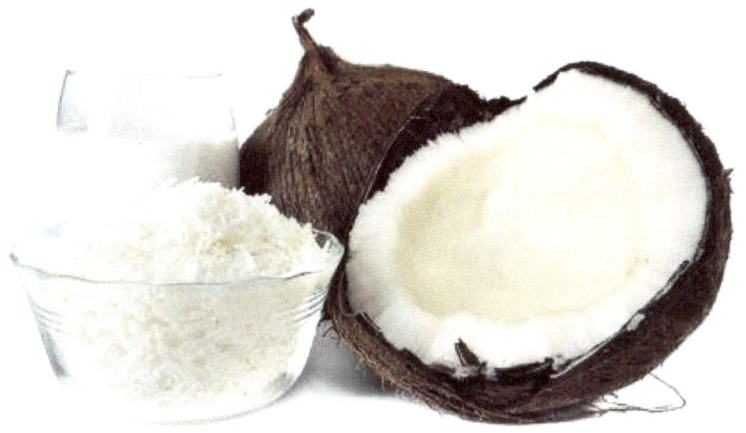

I added dried coconut and fresh coconut and lots of tomatoes to my diet, and placed a tomato pulp poultice on that area for the past three nights. The next morning I washed my face with cold water and absolutely no soap. I am very pleased to see that the possible white marks are diminishing and all within three days. Hooray. I intend to have my skin back uniformly dusky and will continue with this tomato patch as long as it takes.

Okra

Just imagine jambalaya or gumbo without okra. Okra has long been known as a binding item in a number of soups and liquid delicacies and that is why it is rarely eaten as a fried vegetable. Boiling okra is going to make it soggy and wet and quite unpleasant looking. That is why it is always added to a number of ingredients, so that the end product does not look sticky and gummy type.

When I told some of my Creole friends that they could not keep watching their weight, if they continued eating lots of okra, they looked at me with frank disbelief. Not many people know that okra/also known as ladyfingers is capable of helping you put on lots of weight. However, I have the natural antidote for this, especially if you love okra like I do.

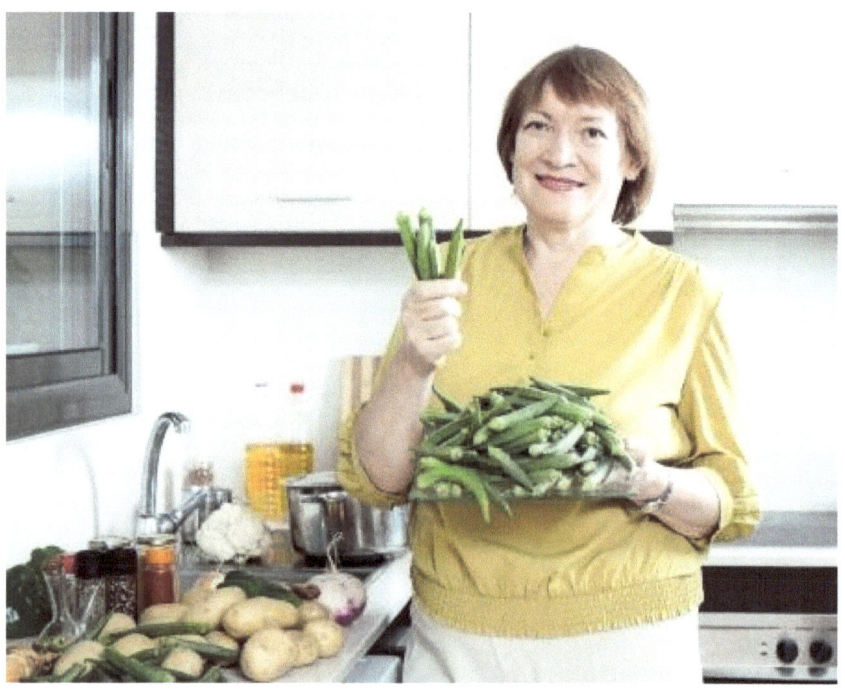

Just cook it with one teaspoonful of cumin seeds and a touch of asafetida. You need about half a pinch of asafetida, which is going to give the dish an onion -like flavor. And you are going to stay slim as ever, even though you eat jambalaya, spicy fried okra, gumbo or any other delicious and nourishing dishes.

Do not wash the okra, before you cut it. Just clean them by rubbing with a wet cloth. Washing brings out the stickiness and you are going to have sticky strands of okra sticking to your knife and fingers when you chop up the pieces.

Potatoes

There is a possibly apocryphal story about the great Mogul Emperor who built the Taj Mahal. His son had put his ailing father under house arrest, after declaring him incompetent enough to rule. So his father was imprisoned in Agra Fort, where he could see the Taj Mahal from his window.

And popular lore says that his son asked his father to name one vegetable and one Grain which he would be given to eat. The father immediately said potatoes and for the grain, he said black gram. Thanks to this choice, his cook could make an amazing new variety of delicacies with potatoes, roasted, baked, mashed, fried, with black gram bread and patties. [1]

The only problem with potatoes is that they are fattening. They should never be eaten raw. They are the best filling food which you can eat, full of carbohydrates and fats. They also happen to be easy to digest, and that is why in the East, old people who need more fat content are given lots of potatoes to eat.

My father stopped eating potatoes in the early 50s, because he said he had had it to the brim with six years of potatoes at engineering college. He was studying in a desert area, where they were absolutely no greens available. So it was potatoes in the morning potatoes in the evening, potatoes at suppertime.

---

[1] I know that this story is imaginary, because the Moguls knew what was due to royalty and even if the Emperor was imprisoned, his family would make sure that he would be treated like an Emperor, and get whatever he wish for, except freedom. It was a matter of *noblesse oblige*. Besides, eating just potatoes and black gram without any other vegetables or proteins would have killed off Shah Jahan through starvation and malnutrition. However, the Emperor survived eight years of imprisonment and illness. Besides, the Emperor was being taken care of by his daughter Jahan- Ara who was later given the title of Empress of Princesses by her brother after their father's death.

When he got out of college with his two engineering Degrees, he promised himself that he would never eat potatoes again under any guise, garb, or excuse. And that is why he stayed as thin as a lathe throughout his life. One could not get any carbohydrates on a diet made up of just meat, bread, eggs and cheese. No vegetables, no fruit. He survived on this not so healthy diet for the next 40 years. When he reached his 80s, I could see that he was suffering from no fat and tried to persuade him to eat some potatoes. He would not. He still does not.

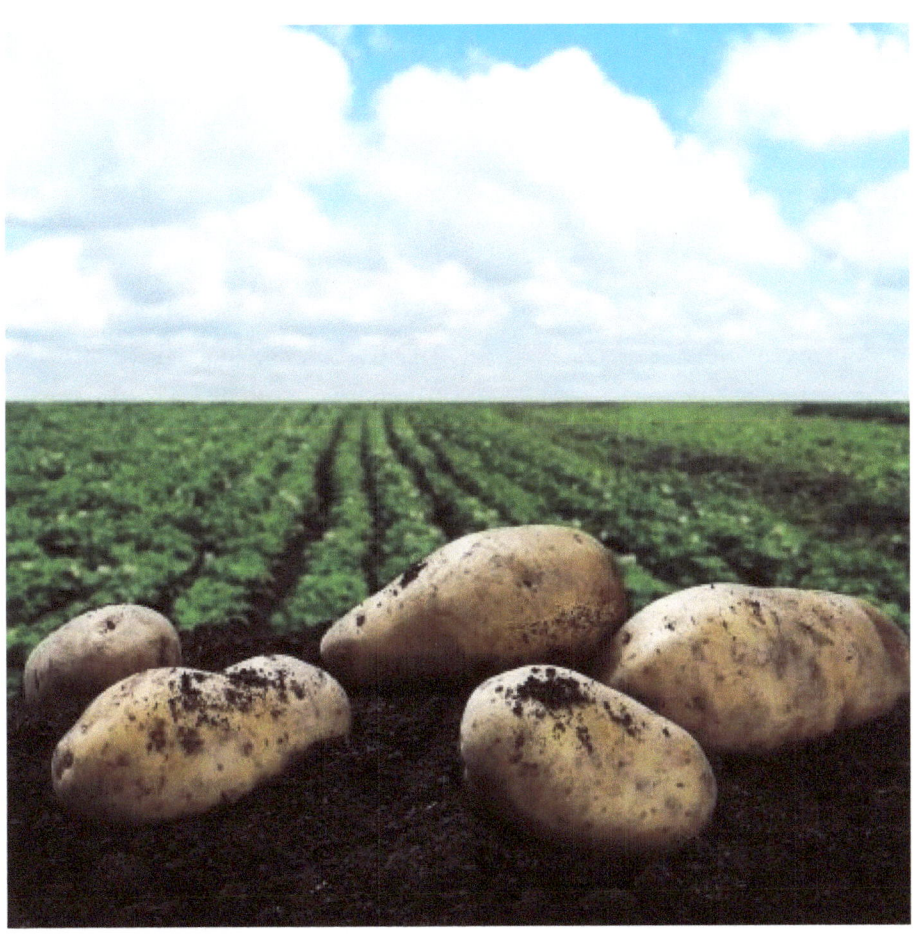

Sad, because he is missing out on one of the most delicious foods given to us by nature.

Acidity

Here is an acidity cure with potatoes. Roast two potatoes, and mash with a little bit of rock salt, cumin seeds, and powdered pepper. Add a little bit of lemon juice on top of this mixture, and eat. You are going to see your stomach clearing up in a little while.

I did not know that this was an acidity cure, because I used to eat this mixture, just for fun, especially with lots of lemon juice added. But then I never suffered from heartburn or acidity ever before and I would not suffer it, in the future.

Potatoes for Burns

It has been known since ancient times that potatoes are the best cure for burns, especially when there is no doctor around. Just put the affected area under cold running water for about 10 to 15 minutes. Get somebody to grate some potatoes in the meanwhile. After 10 minutes, apply the grated potatoes on that area, and cover with a clean cloth. I saw this being done in a jungle area, where there was no hospital around and I did not have any ointment around when one of my friends got burnt in the campfire.

The guide immediately dipped her hand into the cold water of the stream running nearby, while he told the cook to grate some potatoes. That juice and the pulp was applied on the burns and bandaged. We were there for one week and each day we saw those burns healing up whenever the bandages were opened. Every morning, a fresh application of these grated potatoes was done.

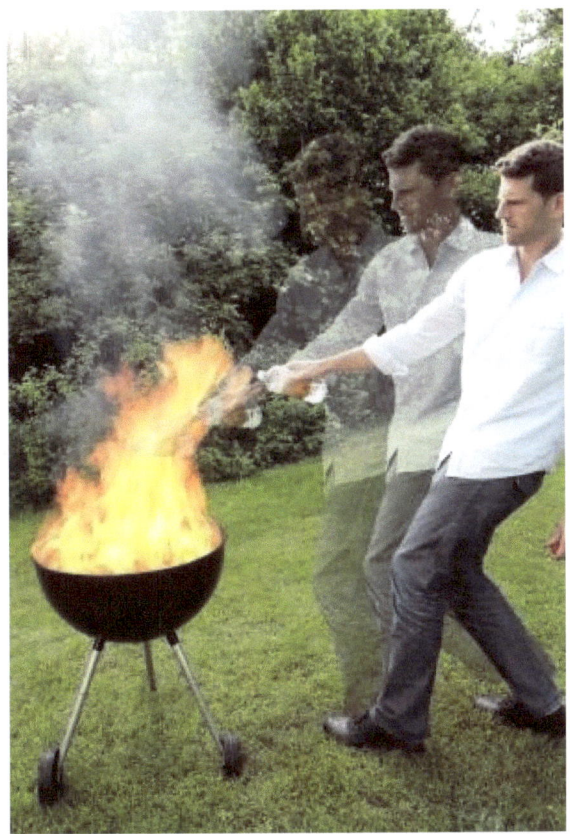

You may want to try it for the next time you burn yourself in the kitchen, and there is no medical aid around.

Potatoes for Eyesight

I found this recipe in a small village hidden somewhere in the mountains where a wise man made sure that the elders of the village never suffered from cataract or from blurred vision. He ground in raw potato on a stone, and removed the juice. This juice was applied on the eyeball to prevent the formation of a cataract as well as to get rid of any blurriness. This was done every day until the vision cleared up perfectly. It would take two months to clear up any potential cataract and blurred vision.

Cabbages

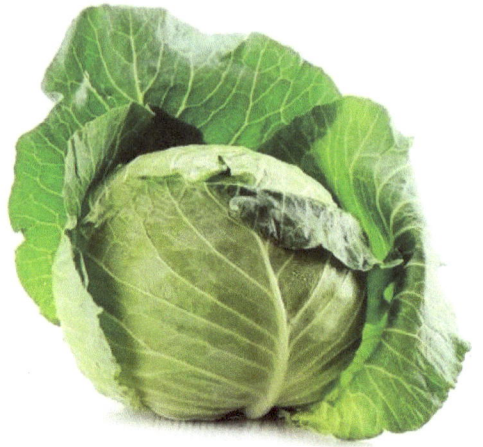

If you are feeling lethargic, make up a salad of tomatoes, cabbages, spinach and drink it down with milk. This is going to give you all the essential minerals necessary to keep you bright eyed and bushy tailed. Apart from cabbages, cauliflowers, and knolkhols also belong to the same family, but for medical purposes, cabbages are considered more efficient, effective and suitable. Thanks to the amount of sulfur present in cabbages, they keep your system healthy. But cabbages are capable of producing flatulence which can be counteracted with adding cumin seeds, tomatoes, and spices to the mixture.

Use any preferred spices, including cinnamon, pepper, cardamom, chili peppers, bishops weed and aniseed. The more spices you put in cabbages, the more they counteract its flatulence creating effect.

Radishes

I asked an elderly acquaintance the reason how he kept healthy, even when he was in his 80s, and his answer was that this was because of the number of radishes he ate. According to me, eating radishes was a definite no-no, thanks to their tendency of causing lots of body odor. That was because of the high percentage of protein in the radishes.

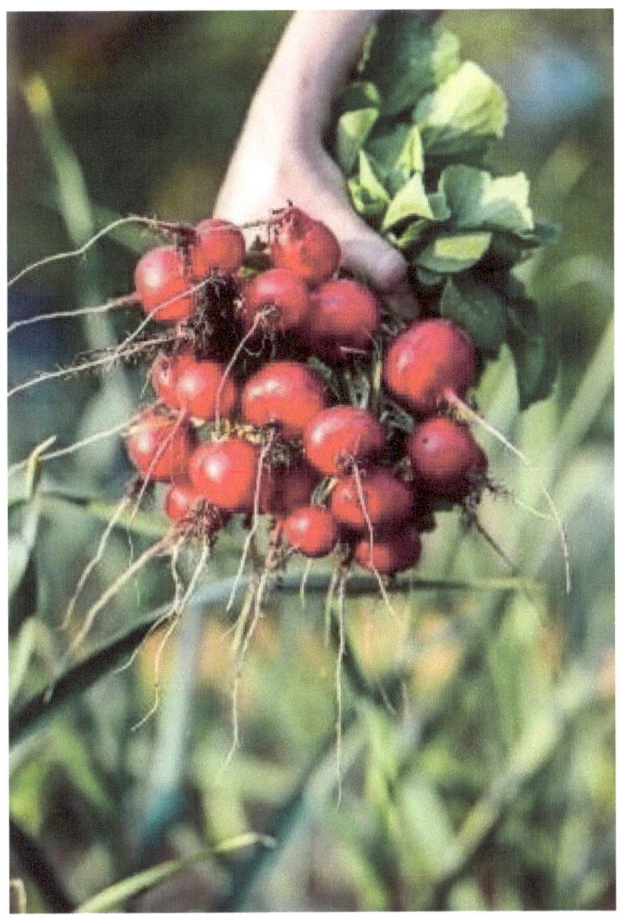

But here is a tip. Do not remove radishes from your daily diet, just because you are worried about bad breath and bad body odor. After you eat radishes, just take a teaspoonful of molasses/jaggery, or half a teaspoonful of any seeds, coriander seeds, or a few mint leaves. You can eat any of these items, whichever you have at hand. This is going to get rid of the body odor as well as radish breath problem.

Jaundice

If you are suffering from jaundice, all you have to do is take some fresh radish leaves, and mix it up with radish juice, 30 g of each is going to do you very fine. Now add a little bit of brown sugar or molasses, to this mixture and drink this up morning and evening. You are going to be cured within 20 – 25 days.

Apart from the radish juice, the usage of molasses here is justified. Sugarcane juice is extremely good for jaundice. So concentrated sugarcane juice in the form of molasses is going to help cure you of jaundice.

Fenugreek

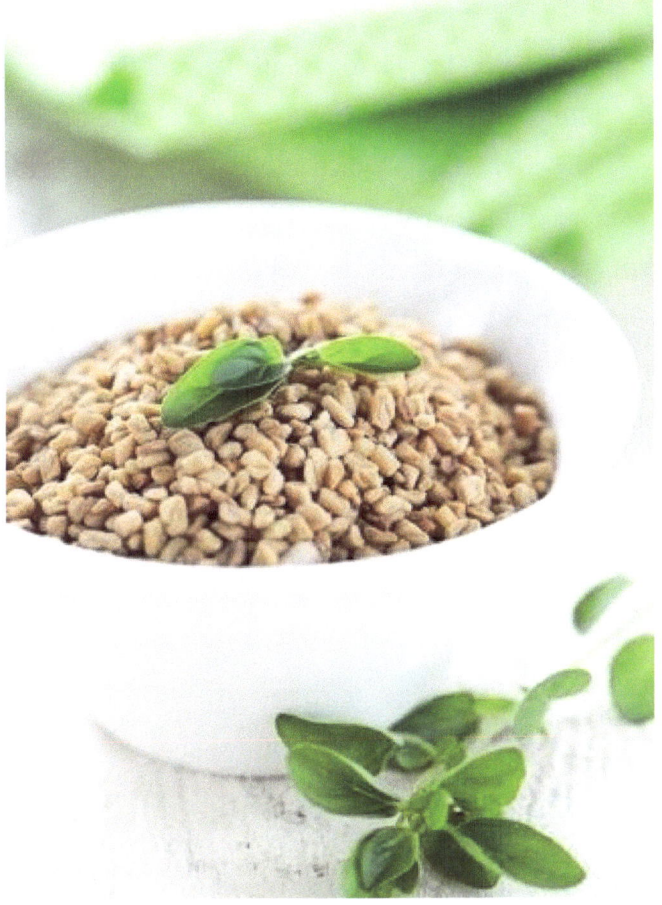

Fenugreek seeds have long been used to cure a number of ailments, and their leaves are also a delicious vegetable addition to your diet. In many parts of the world, these leaves are eaten mixed up with spinach and tomatoes, especially in the winter. This combination is extremely good for your health.

In fact, eating fenugreek in the winter is extremely good for your body because it generates heat, especially when it is freezing out there. Apart from this, you are going to get a number of trace minerals necessary for your body like sulfur, iron and manganese in fresh fenugreek leaves.

Fenugreek seeds have been known to be anti-flatulent curatives because they prevent the formation of toxic flatulence in your stomach during the digestive process. Here is one tip which you may want to utilize, especially if you have stopped eating beans because of their flatulent qualities. Just add one teaspoonful of fenugreek seeds, in the beans, while cooking. You may also want to add some soya seeds to make this mixture even more digestible, and also to prevent fat buildup. It is surprising that so many people who are worried about their weight or their fat content have not tried out a mixture of fenugreek seeds and soya seeds in the food they eat.

Carrots

Carrots are an excellent source of vitamin A. Apart from giving you strong jawbones and excellent teeth, when you chew them, they have also been used for millenniums to get rid of a large number of ailments.

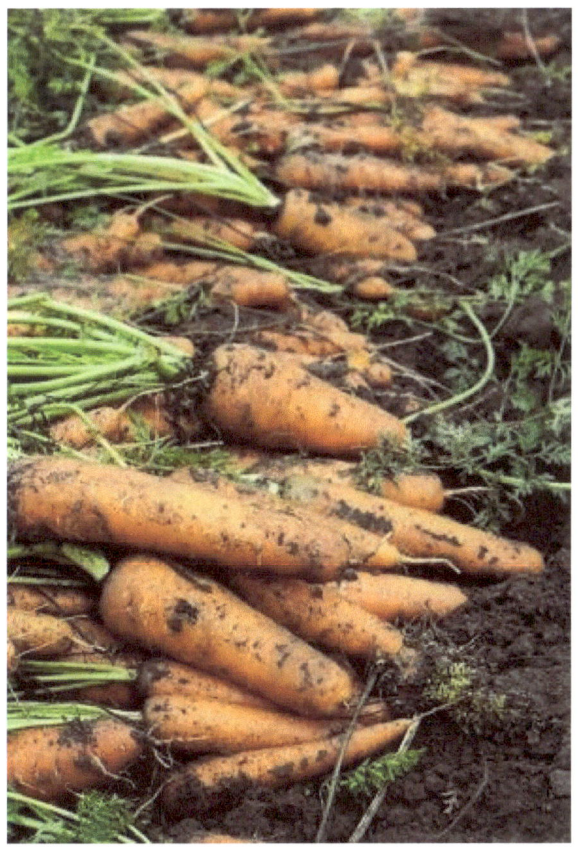

Migraine

If you are suffering from chronic migraine, or even migraine triggered off due to stress or eating lots of chocolates, – my migraine attacks used to be triggered off with just the flash of a camera; I remember a terrible instance, when I had a horrible attack in a palace which I was visiting with my fellow classmates from Business School. All of them took out their cameras and began clicking the walls, which were embedded with glass. Millions of reflected surfaces, and camera flashes flashing. I was hors de combat for 48 hours.

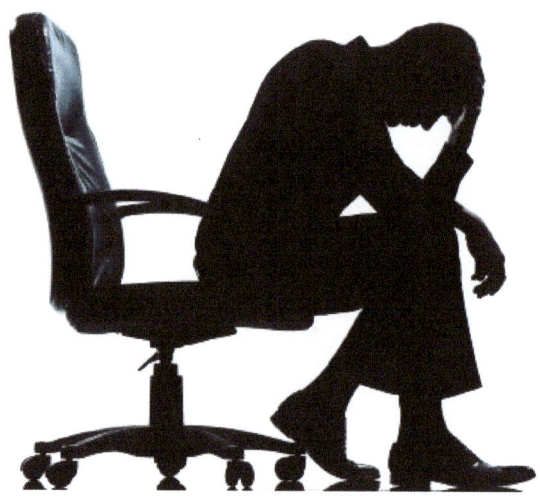

Oh, this headache!

At that time I did not know about this particular migraine cure and had to deal with Migril and Vasograin with Stemetil to prevent nausea. I could not stir out anywhere without these in my purse.

This cure was told to me by an experienced old naturopath. Just grind some leaves of carrots and heat them up. Allow to cool to lukewarm, and put two drops morning and evening in your ears and in your nostrils. This is going to clear up your system amazingly and get rid of all those migraine attacks.

When asked him how long I had to do this, he said "as long as it takes". As far as I know, one of his patients did this for one month and she has not had a migraine attack for the last seven years.

Try it out for one month, and see if you suffer from any attack again.

Aubergines/eggplants/Brinjals

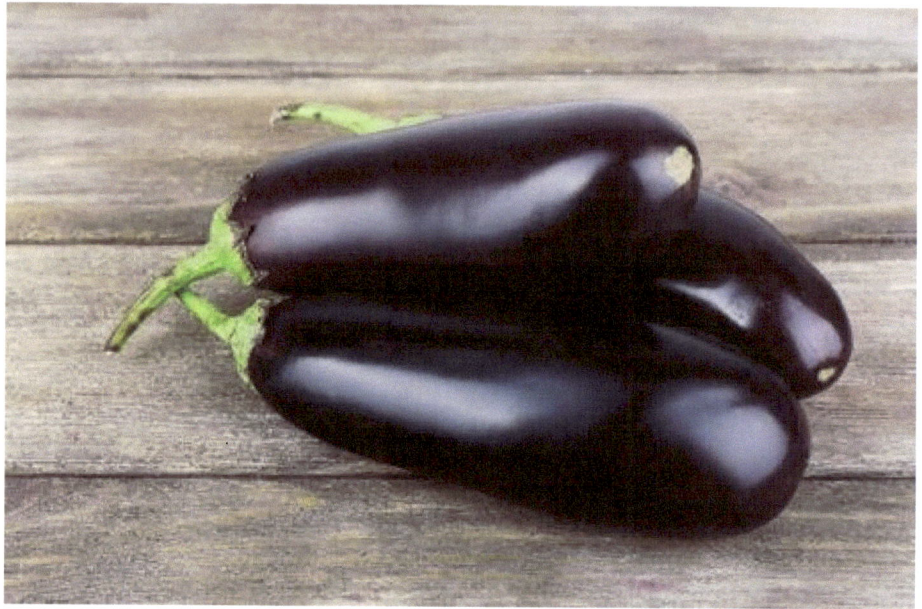

Many people do not enjoy eating aubergines, because according to them, they are so bland and tasteless. What they do not know is that roasted Aubergines eaten every day have been known to cure **piles**. Also, people who are suffering from **insomnia** just need to add some aubergines to their diet, and they are going to find themselves sleeping naturally, and long.

Here is one amusing incident, I must tell you about some of the curative properties of aubergines, which I found just by chance. I was roasting them on the gas stove, along with some chopped pieces and the burning skin and the roasting pieces were emitting thick smoke. I was suffering from ear ache that day, and I just happened to place my ear in the path of the smoke. The earache vanished! I do not know whether it was because of the hot "fomentation"by the smoke, or by something in the roasting aubergines. After that, I just cleaned out my ear with a little bit of hydrogen peroxide, and no pain in the ear since then. So next time you suffer from some sort of yearly, or even toothache with that particular area swollen, try seeing the effect of smoking aubergines to cure you. Incidentally, if you are suffering from hair loss, begin eating more eggplants. You are soon going to find your hair growing in a healthy manner.

If you want to fry them, I would suggest a method with which you do not need to use so much of cooking fat or oil. Just cut them into small pieces and sprinkle salt on them. Then leave them for about half an hour and fry them in minimal oil. This is an excellent vegetable for people who want to lose weight.

Flatulence Cure

If you are suffering from flatulence, all you have to do is chop up some aubergines and cook them with a little bit of garlic and asafetida. Eat it with the rest of your meal, as if you are eating this as a chutney. I found a friend of mine making a bottle of this, and preserving it in her fridge to be fed to the rest of her family over the next three days as a chutney accompaniment to foods causing possible flatulence like cabbage, beans, etc.

Conclusion

This book has given you plenty of interesting information on how you can keep healthy with lots of fresh vegetables in your diet. Apart from this, you have also learned some natural beauty tips, which are going to keep you looking good throughout your life.

So add vegetables to your diet right now, Live Long and Prosper!

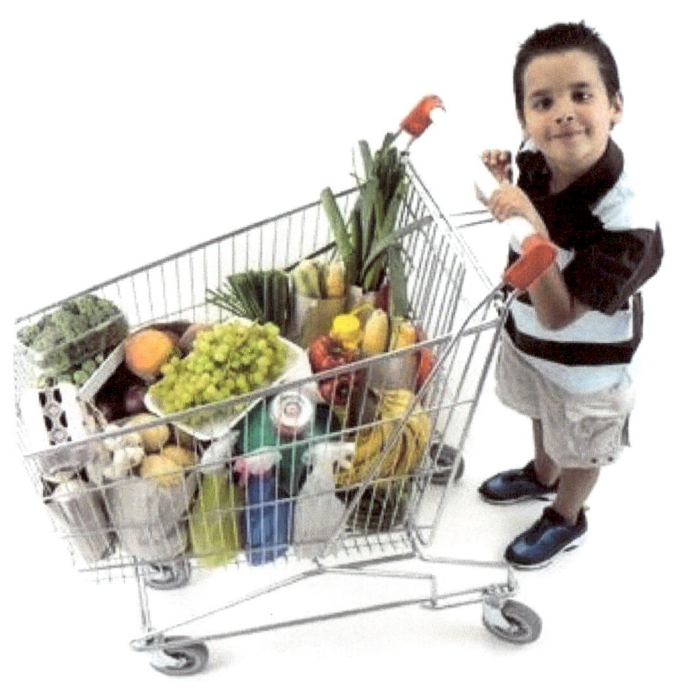

Author Bio

Dueep Jyot Singh is a Management and IT Professional who managed to gather Postgraduate qualifications in Management and English and Degrees in Science, French and Education while pursuing different enjoyable career options like being an hospital administrator, IT,SEO and HRD Database Manager/ trainer, movie , radio and TV scriptwriter, theatre artiste and public speaker, lecturer in French, Marketing and Advertising, ex-Editor of Hearts On Fire (now known as Solstice) Books Missouri USA, advice columnist and cartoonist, publisher and Aviation School trainer, ex-moderator on Medico.in, banker, student councilor ,travelogue writer … among other things!

One fine morning, she decided that she had enough of killing herself by Degrees and went back to her first love -- writing. It's more enjoyable! She already has 48 published academic and 14 fiction- in- different- genre books under her belt.

When she is not designing websites or making Graphic design illustrations for clients , she is browsing through old bookshops hunting for treasures, of which she has an enviable collection – including R.L. Stevenson, O.Henry, Dornford Yates, Maurice Walsh, De Maupassant, Victor Hugo, Sapper, C.N. Williamson, "Bartimeus" and the crown of her collection- Dickens "The Old Curiosity Shop," and "Martin Chuzzlewit" and so on… Just call her "Renaissance Woman" - collecting herbal remedies, acting like Universal Helping Hand/Agony Aunt, or escaping to her dear mountains for a bit of exploring, collecting herbs and plants, and trekking.

Check out some of the other JD-Biz Publishing books

Gardening Series on Amazon

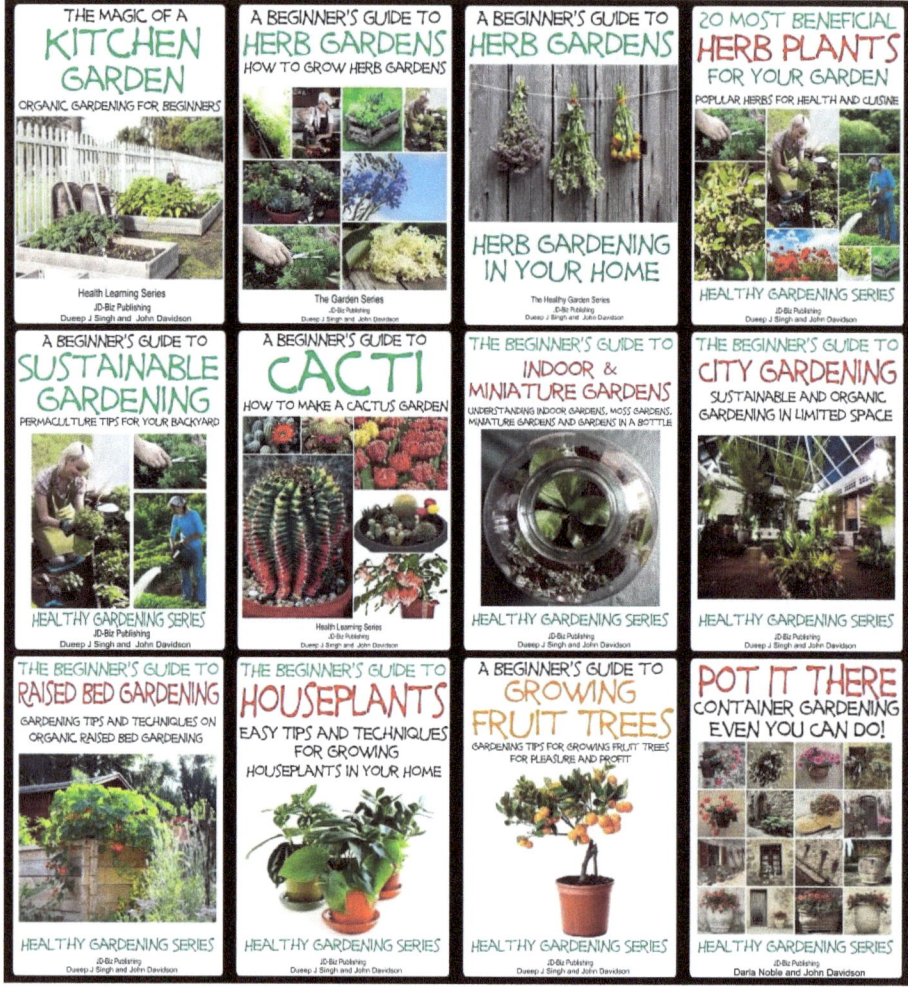

Download Free Books!

http://MendonCottageBooks.com

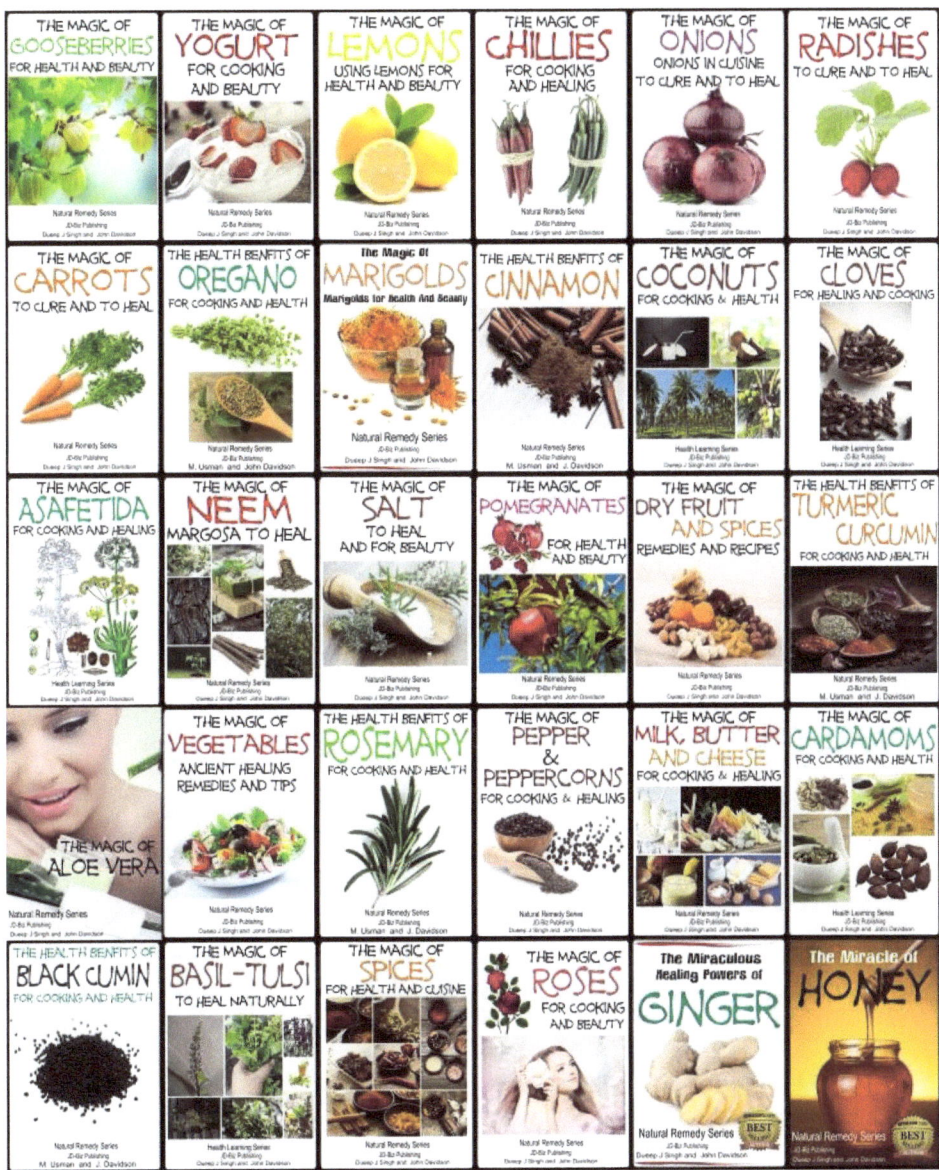

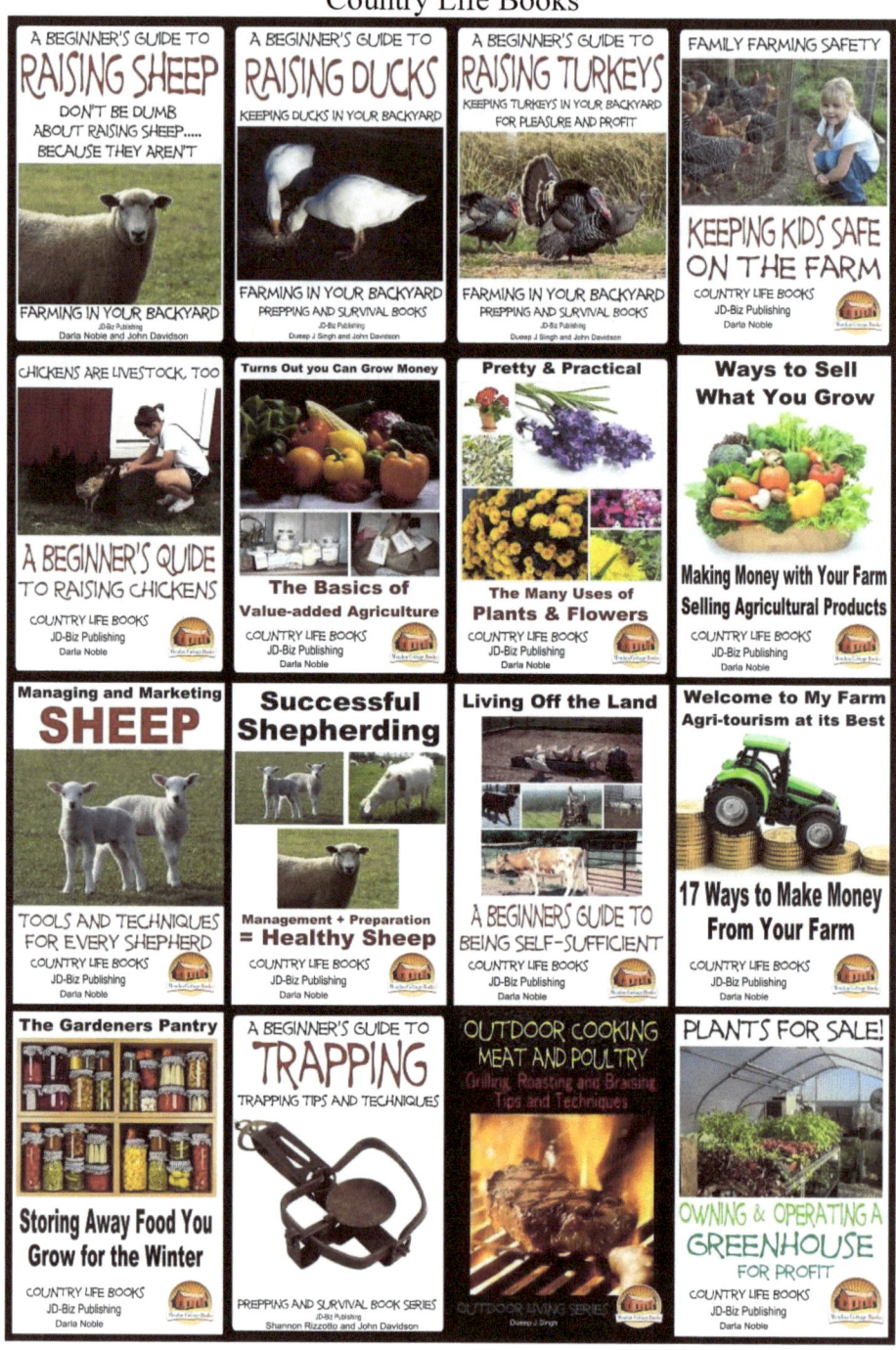

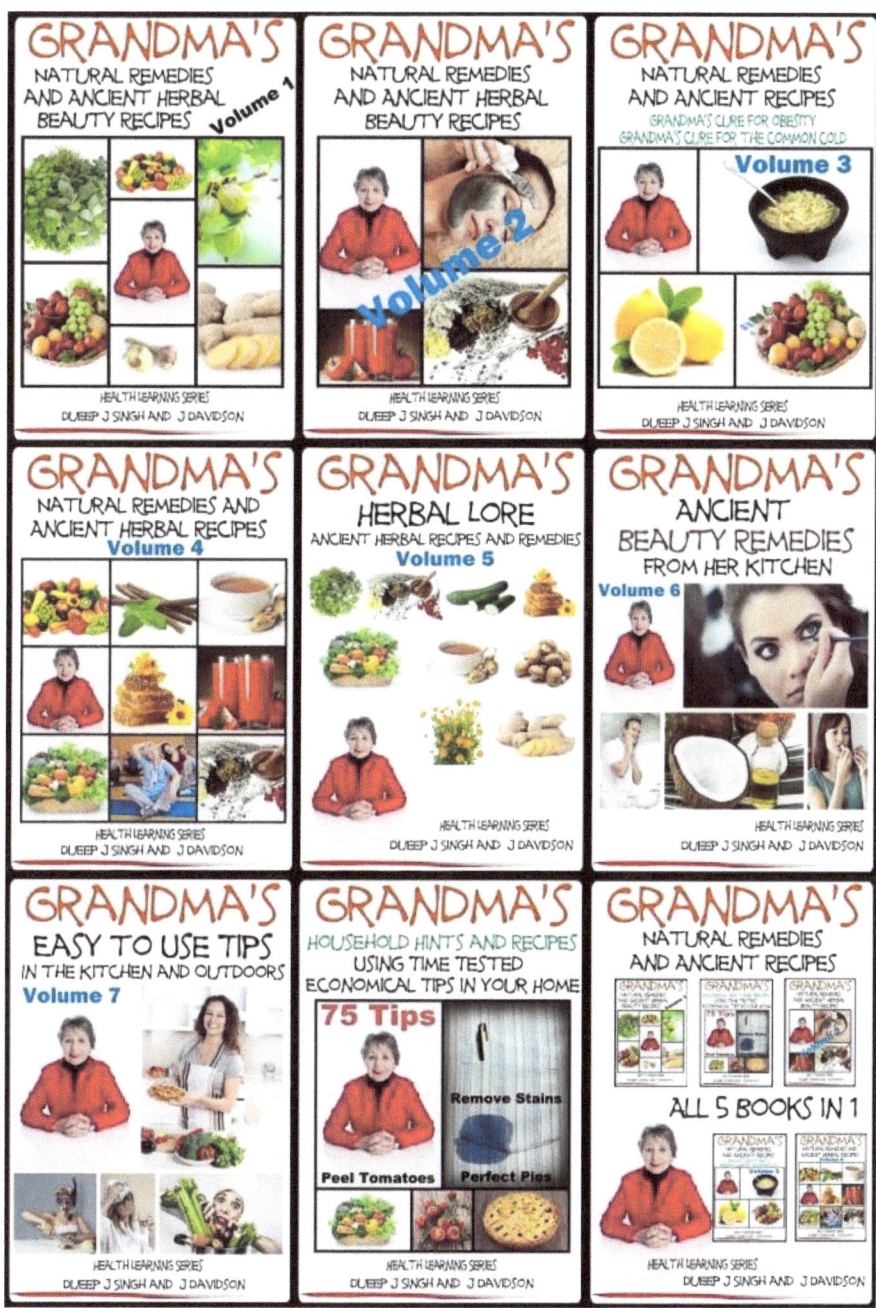

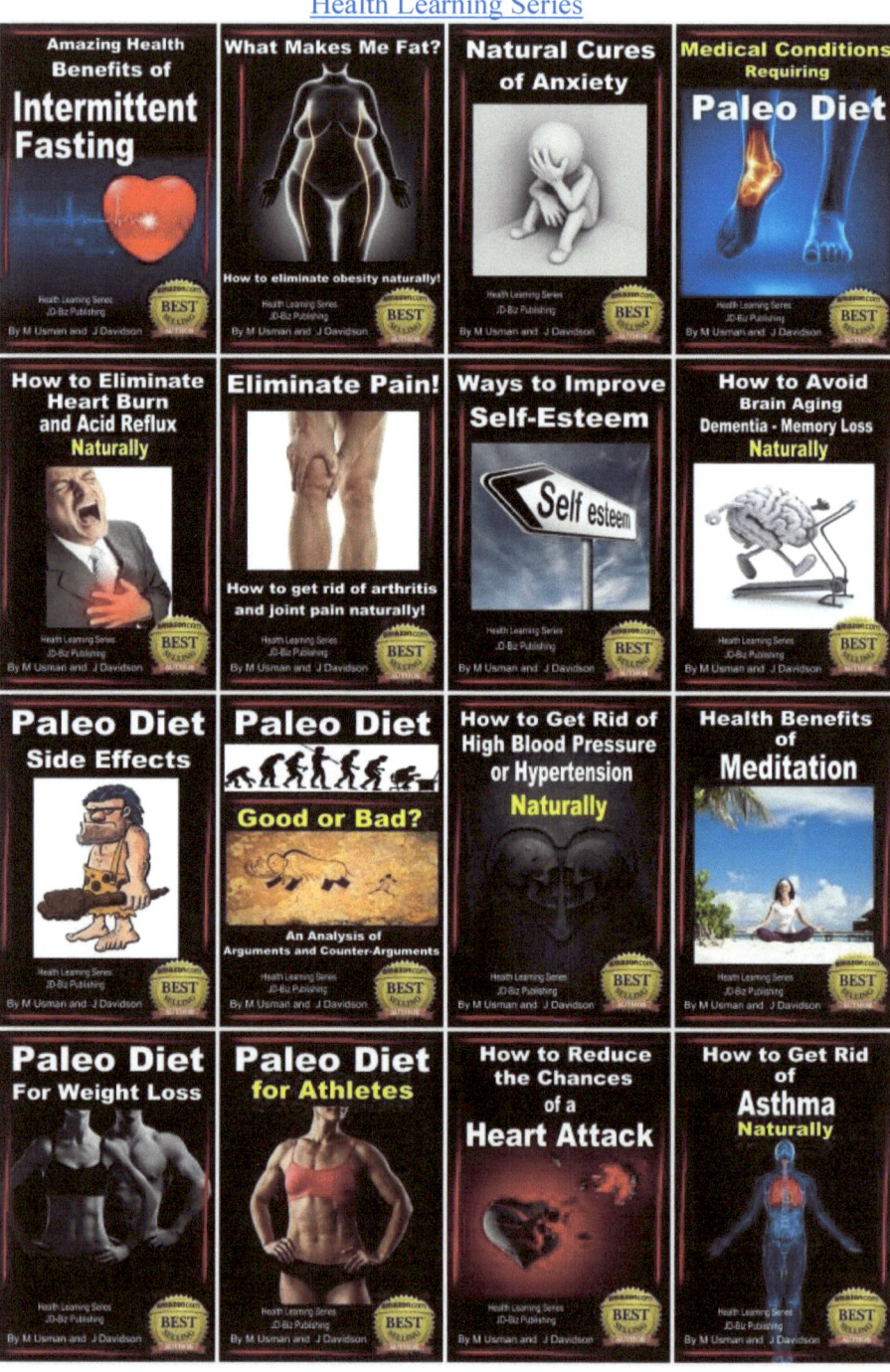

Amazing Animal Book Series

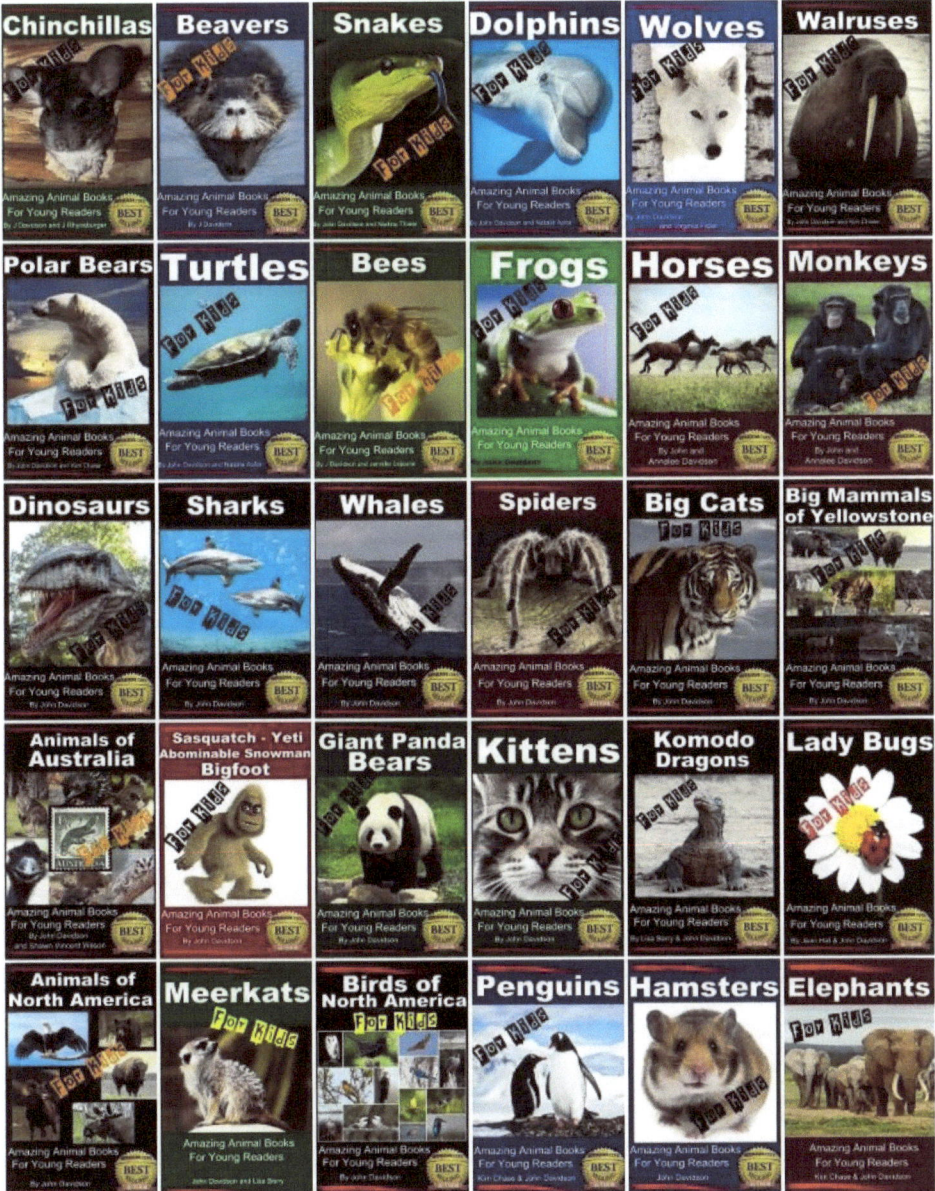

Learn To Draw Series

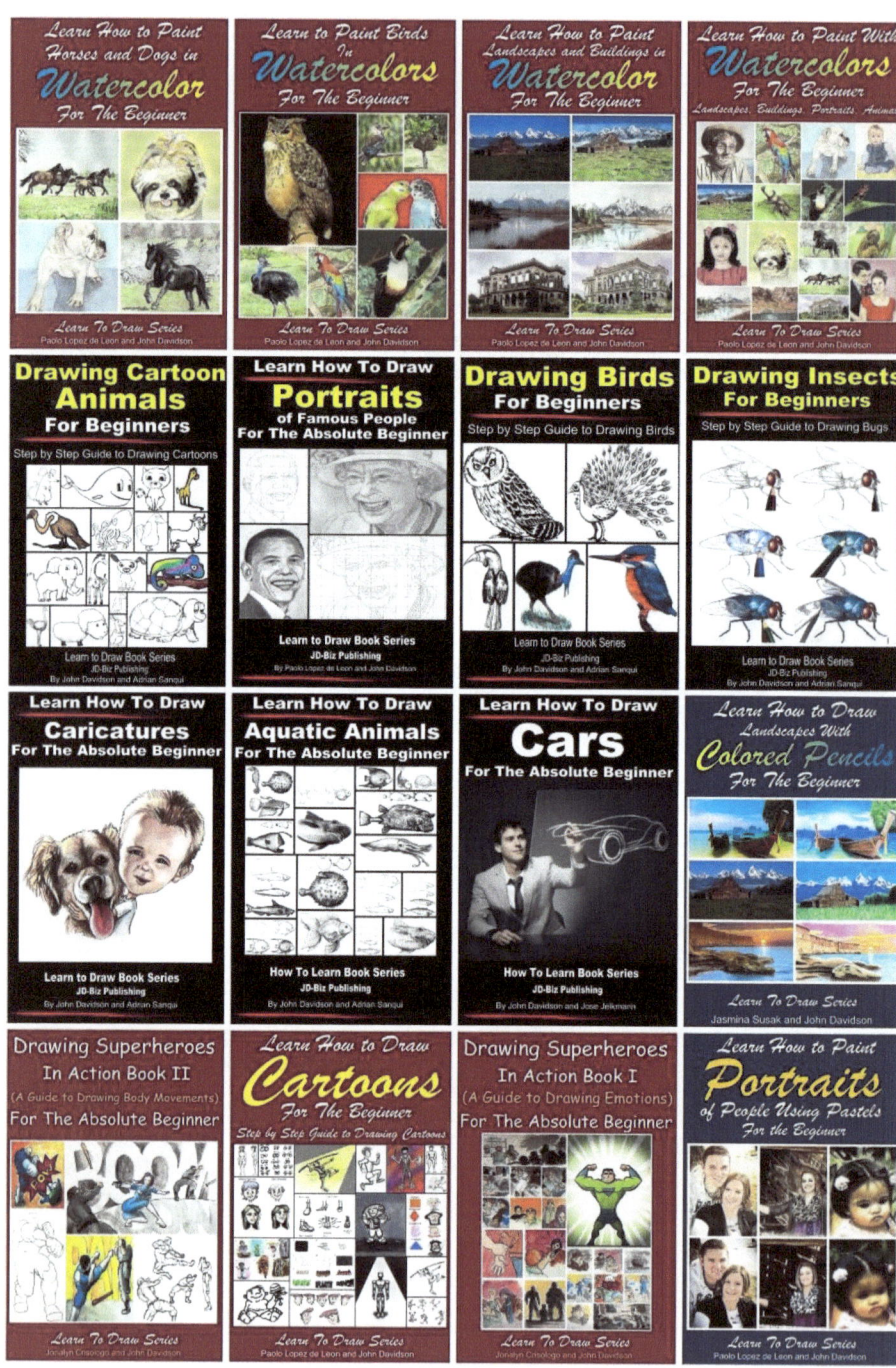

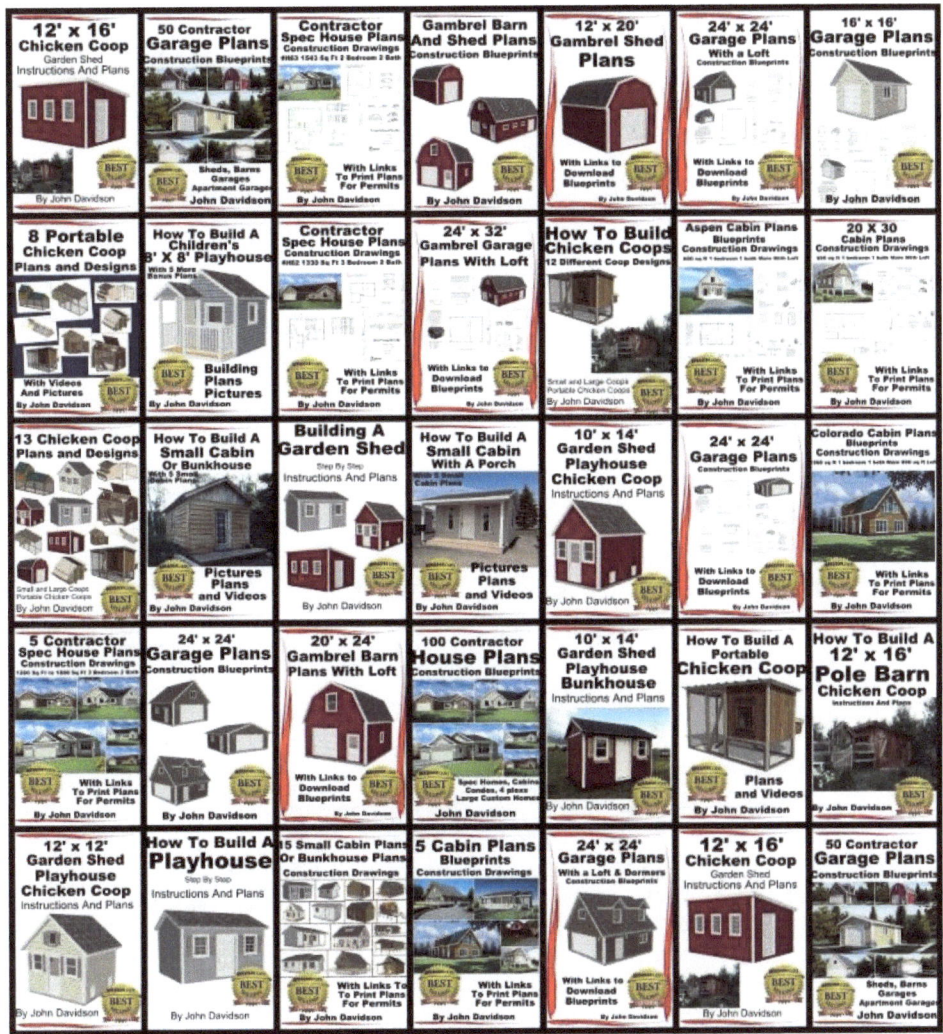

Entrepreneur Book Series

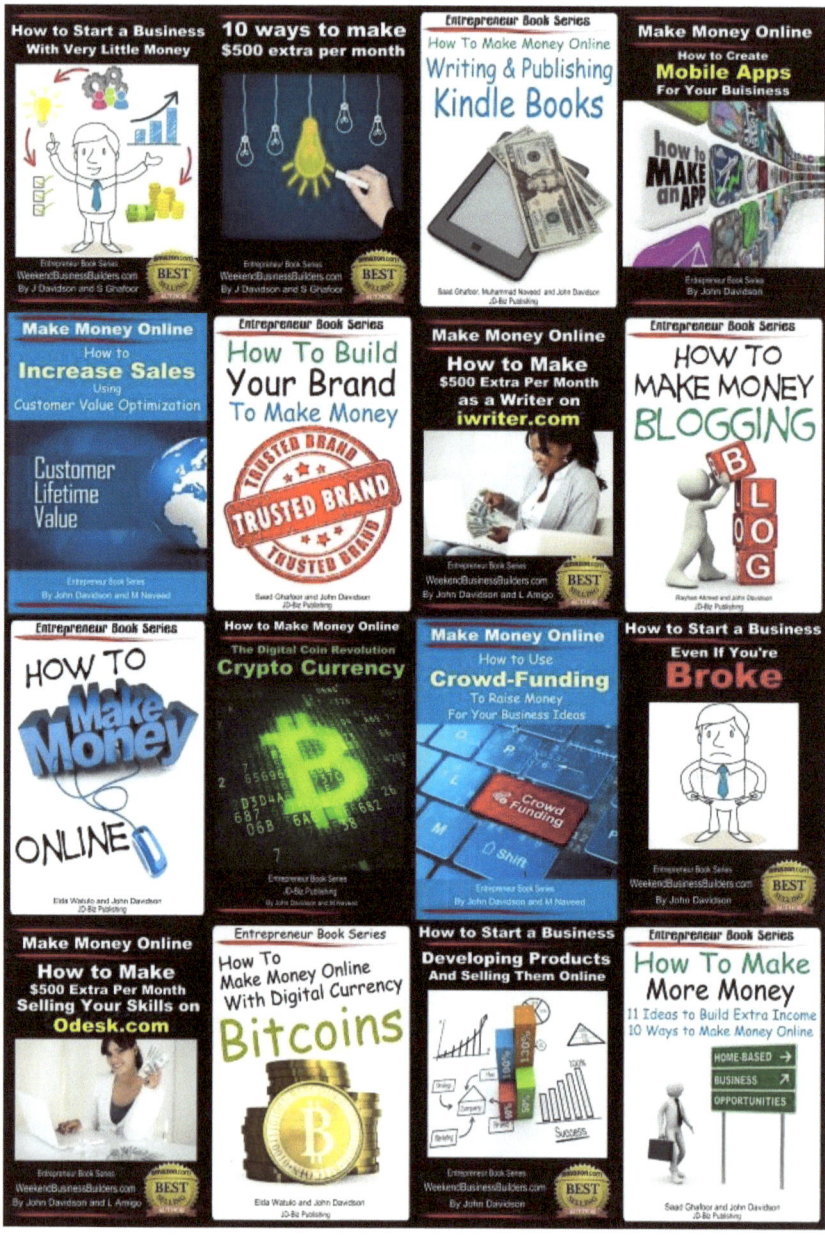

Our books are available at

1. Amazon.com

2. Barnes and Noble

3. Itunes

4. Kobo

5. Smashwords

6. Google Play Books

Download Free Books!

http://MendonCottageBooks.com

Publisher

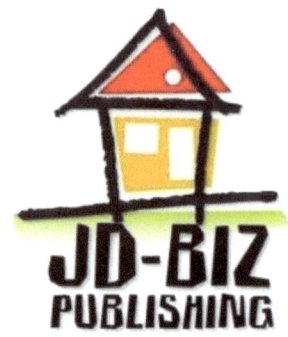

JD-Biz Corp

P O Box 374

Mendon, Utah 84325

http://www.jd-biz.com/

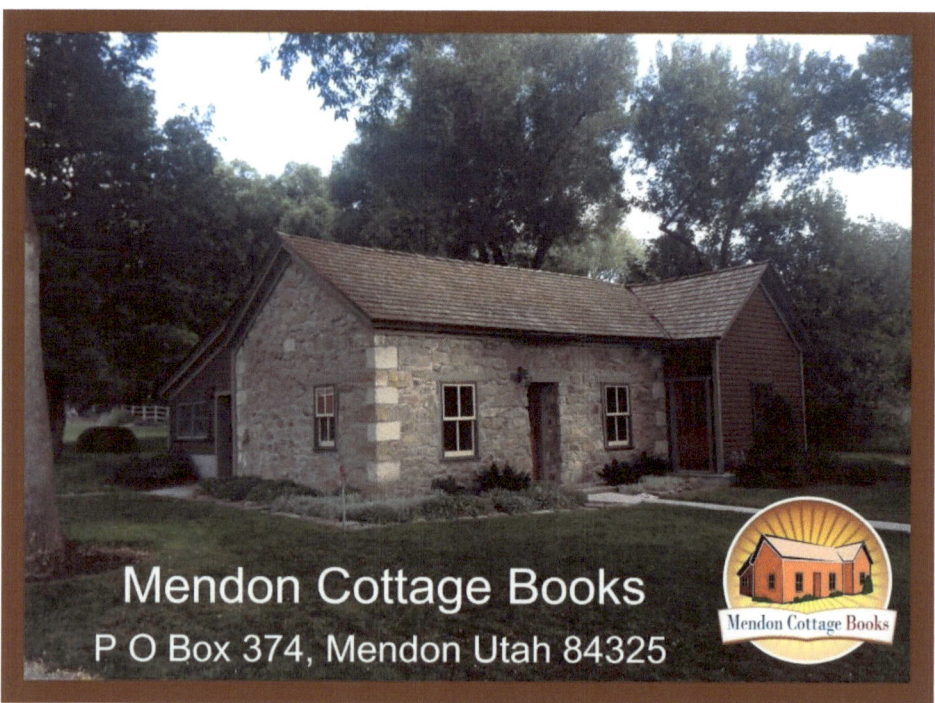